KINETICS AND DYNAMICS OF INTRAVENOUS ANESTHETICS

DEVELOPMENTS IN
CRITICAL CARE MEDICINE AND ANESTHESIOLOGY

Volume 26

The titles published in this series are listed at the end of this volume.

KINETICS AND DYNAMICS
OF
INTRAVENOUS ANESTHETICS

by

GERARLD M. WOERLEE M.B., B.S. (W. Aust.), F.F.A.R.C.S. (Lond.)

Consultant Anesthesiologist,
Rijnoord Hospital,
Alphen aan den Rijn, The Netherlands

Springer-Science+Business Media, B.V.

Library of Congress Cataloging-in-Publication Data

Woerlee, Gerald M.
    Kinetics and dynamics of intravenous anesthetics / by Gerald M.
Woerlee.
        p.   cm. -- (Developments in critical care medicine, and
anesthesiology ; 26)
    Includes index.

    1. Intravenous anesthetics--Pharmacokinetics.   I. Title.
II. Series.
RD85.I6W63   1992
617.9'62--Jc20   91-45063

ISBN 978-94-017-4097-5   ISBN 978-0-585-28009-7 (eBook)
DOI 10.1007/978-0-585-28009-7

Printed on acid-free paper

Contents

Contents

Acknowledgements

I wish to express my gratitude to, and acknowledge the invaluable aid of Professor Dr. P.J. Hennis, Professor of Anesthesiology in the University Hospital of Groningen, Groningen, the Netherlands, for his constructive criticism and tireless review of the manuscript, in spite of exceptionally busy personal and professional circumstances. Dr C. Brandon-Bravo is another colleague to whom special thanks are due. He too found time to read, and provide valuable insights and criticism on the text. I also wish to extend my thanks to Professor Dr. J. Spierdijk, head of Department, together with the other members of the staff, and of course the residents of the Department of Anesthesiology, University Hospital of Leiden, Leiden, the Netherlands, for the many pleasurable years in which I worked and taught, and myself learnt to appreciate the insights into drug use provided by the sciences discussed in this book.

Last, but not least I wish to acknowledge the patience, encouragement and sound advice provided by my wife Madhuri.

G.M. Woerlee,
Oegstgeest,
October 1991.

Introduction

Definitions are required so that all parties communicating with each other can actually understand what is being communicated. So without any apology whatsoever, I will begin this book with two important definitions which define the subject matter of this book with some precision.

Pharmacokinetics is the study of the uptake, distribution, and elimination of drugs, while *pharmacodynamics* is the study of the effects of drugs in relation to their tissue concentrations.

The last ten years have seen an enormous upsurge of interest in the pharmacokinetics and pharmacodynamics of anesthetic drugs, evidence of a growing appreciation among anesthesiologists of the practical utility of the insights provided by these sciences. This book has been written in response to a perceived requirement by anesthesiologists for a basic text explaining pharmacokinetic and pharmacodynamic principles in a manner which is specifically oriented to the daily experience and training of anesthesiologists, and which provides insights and methods which are readily applicable to daily clinical practice.

The discussion in this book confines itself exclusively to the kinetics and dynamics of drugs administered by the intravenous route. Why only the intravenous route? Very simply because it is a route which is most commonly used to administer drugs in current anesthetic practice.

Tissue drug concentrations, and the effects that drugs exert can be calculated using pharmacokinetic and pharmacodynamic principles. This makes it possible to predict the effects of any given drug at any time after administration. However, it must be said that anesthesia can be practiced to a very high standard by practitioners who are in total ignorance of anything to do with the formal study of the pharmacokinetic and pharmacodynamic properties of the drugs that they use, except knowledge of such factors as the dosages required, and the usual magnitude and duration of action for such doses. This is as true today as it ever was, even when one considers the administration of modern drugs. Such empirical use of drugs will always remain because it is simple and eminently practical. This begs the question of why anyone should then wish to learn anything at all about pharmacokinetics and pharmacodynamics.

The answer to the above question is best illustrated with a true anecdote. During a scientific meeting of the Netherlands Association of Anesthesiologists in 1983, a lecture was given on the 3-compartment kinetic-dynamic model of pancuronium. This lecture was accompanied by double projection of beautiful multicolored slides replete with complicated equations and graphs. At the end of the lecture the audience was given the opportunity to ask questions. An anesthesiologist stood up. This was a middle aged man who had practiced anesthesiology in a busy general hospital for many years. He asked, "I have administered pancuronium to my patients for many years. I always give every adult patient four milligrams of pancuronium regardless of sex, weight or age. It always works well. After listening to your lecture I am in some confusion as to whether I am administering pancuronium in the correct manner. How do you administer pancuronium?" The speaker replied, "Oh, I also give every adult patient four milligrams of pancuronium too." A gale of laughter swept over the audience.

Now the point of this wonderful story is that both persons were correct. The anesthesiologist from the busy general hospital had enormous practical experience in the use of pancuronium. His teachers, as well as his own clinical experience had taught him that four milligrams of pancuronium was an adequate dose for the average adult patient. The lecturer knew that the pharmacokinetic and pharmacodynamic properties of pancuronium were such that four milligrams were sufficient for the average adult patient. Both had arrived at the same answer, four milligrams of pancuronium. All this illustrates is that kinetic-dynamic theory is simply a method of abstractly predicting what can also be empirically determined. However, consider the situation arising should the pancuronium dosage regimen deviate from standard practice. The empirical anesthesiologist will not be able to predict the effect of such a new and untried regimen. However the anesthesiologist who understands the underlying pharmacokinetic and pharmacodynamic theory can make clinically useful predictions. Such predictions are not limited to only one situation, but can be made for any number of situations. This is the power of pharmacokinetic-pharmacodynamic theory. It provides a theoretical basis for every conceivable method of drug use.

Having said all this, it is well worth mentioning that the use of kinetic and dynamic principles have their limitations. The main problem is that current kinetic and dynamic data are all AVERAGE values. So the value of any given kinetic and dynamic parameter is above the average level in some of the persons in any given study population, and below the average level in the rest of that population. This would not be so bad were it not that the variation of such data is often depressingly large. In addition, the study population and circumstances under which a given set of data were derived may be totally different from that of the population and circumstances in which the data are applied. So pharmacokinetics and pharmacodynamics should never be considered as exact sciences at this time. Rather they should be viewed as sciences which provide insights into the way in which drugs are distributed throughout the body, and the relation between drug concentration and effect. Within these limitations it is still possible to make predictions which are clinically useful, as well as to explain the reasons why drugs are used in the way that they are.

The purpose of this book is to teach the reader just such an appreciation of the kinetic and dynamic properties of intravenous anesthetic drugs. This is done using a fivefold approach.

- The basic elements of multicompartment kinetic-dynamic models are explained.

- The relationship between physiology and drug kinetic-dynamic theory is not just discussed in one place, but emphasized throughout the book.

- A new phase in intravenous drug pharmacokinetics is introduced, the "pre-recirculation phase". This explains many of the clinical effects of drugs administered as a single rapid intravenous dose.

- Readers are introduced to an approach to the application of drug kinetics and dynamics to common clinical situations in anesthesia. Many examples using common clinical problems are used to illustrate this approach.

- Causes of variation in drug kinetic parameters encountered in clinical practice are discussed in chapters 7 to 14. This enables the reader to adjust the results of any kinetic-dynamic calculations in the appropriate direction.

The two appendices list the physico-chemical, kinetic and dynamic properties of the most commonly used intravenously administered drugs in anesthesia. This information is readily applied to nearly all kinetic and dynamic calculations.

And finally, the information presented in this book is provided with extensive lists of references so that the reader has entry into what the author considers to be basic source material in these rapidly developing subjects.

Chapter 1

Basic Mathematical Principles

A qualitative appreciation of drug kinetic and dynamic principles has practical clinical uses, but is less useful than when combined with a quantitative understanding of these same principles. Fortunately all anesthesiologists have studied mathematics up to high school level. No more knowledge than this is needed to understand this book. The purpose of this chapter is to review in a brief and very selective manner the mathematical principles required.

The last section of this chapter, and the most important, deals with the basic principles of the mathematical description of pharmacokinetic "compartments". This is a powerful concept which is used in all current drug kinetic and dynamic models. Methods are shown with which the reader can derive and solve equations describing the concentrations of drugs within pharmacokinetic compartments. The reader is requested to read this section as these principles are used in other chapters of this book.

Some parts of this chapter may seem excessively trite and simple to some readers, and the author begs the reader's indulgence for this. Nonetheless it is the author's experience that it is just these topics which cause the most problems to students of pharmacokinetics.

EXPONENTIAL FUNCTIONS

The first topic that will be discussed is that of exponential functions and processes. An appreciation of the properties of exponential functions is basic to the understanding of the kinetics and dynamics of any drug. These properties can nearly always be described using the properties of exponentials. The properties of exponential functions are best learnt using examples.

EXAMPLE 1.1:

Consider a left ventricle which contains no drug. Suddenly blood containing a drug at a concentration of 100 mg/L starts to enter the left ventricle. The concentration of that drug in the left ventricle increases with each successive contraction until it equals 100 mg/L. Drug concentration in the incoming blood is the target concentration (C_{target}). What is the relationship between the cardiac contraction cycle number and drug concentration in the left ventricle?

Basic physiology of the left ventricle

The left ventricle never fully empties during systole. In fact, the stroke volume (SV) of the left ventricle is only 67% = 0.67 of the end-diastolic volume (EDV). This means that the end-systolic volume (ESV) of the left ventricle is 33% = 0.33 of the EDV.

Drug concentration in the left ventricle

Let "n" denote the cardiac cycle number occurring after drug containing blood starts to enter the left ventricle, and "C" denote drug concentration. If the basic physiology described above is taken into account, the amount (M_1) of drug present in the left ventricle at the end of the first diastolic period during which drug containing blood enters is given by the equation below.

$$M_1 = SV.C_{target}$$

Now stroke volume = SV = EDV - ESV, and so the equation above may be changed to;

$$M_1 = C_{target}.EDV - C_{target}.ESV$$

Divide the above equation by the EDV to obtain an equation giving drug concentration in the left ventricle at the end of the first period of diastole that drug containing blood enters.

$$C_1 = C_{target} - C_{target}\frac{ESV}{EDV} = C_{target} - C_{target}.f_x$$

Therefore; C_1 = 100 - 100 x 0.33 = 100(1 - 0.33) = 67 mg/L

Now 67% of the blood volume in the left ventricle is pumped out with each contraction, which means that each successive contraction reduces the magnitude of f_x to 33% of its value in the previous contraction. So the left ventricular drug concentration at the end of the second diastolic period is;

$$C_2 = 100 - 100 \times 0.33 \times 0.33 = 100(1 - 0.33^2) = 89.1 \text{ mg/L}$$

This process is repeated during the third diastolic period, and so;

$$C_3 = 100 - 100 \times 0.33^2 \times 0.33 = 100(1 - 0.33^3) = 96.4 \text{ mg/L}$$

This means that a general equation describing the diastolic drug concentration in the left ventricle at any cardiac cycle number after drug starts to enter is given by equation 1.1.

$$C_n = 100(1 - 0.33^n) \qquad (1.1)$$

Fractional change of drug concentration per contraction

The fractional change of drug concentration in the left ventricle with each successive cardiac concentration is shown below.

- Fractional change C_0 to C_1 = $\dfrac{C_1 - C_0}{C_{target} - C_0}$ = $\dfrac{67 - 0}{100 - 0}$ = 0.67

- Fractional change C_1 to C_2 = $\dfrac{C_2 - C_1}{C_{target} - C_1}$ = $\dfrac{89.1 - 67}{100 - 67}$ = 0.67

- Fractional change C_2 to C_3 = $\dfrac{C_3 - C_2}{C_{target} - C_2}$ = $\dfrac{96.4 - 89.1}{100 - 89.1}$ = 0.67

From the above it is evident that the fractional change of drug concentration in the left ventricle with each successive cardiac contraction is a constant fraction of the DIFFERENCE between the existing drug concentration and the target drug concentration. This is a typical feature of exponential change.

EXAMPLE 1.2:

A drug is injected very rapidly into the left ventricle, and after mixing with the blood there, the drug concentration is 100 mg/L. The incoming blood contains no drug, and so the drug concentration in the left ventricle will now decrease with each successive cardiac cycle. What is the relationship between cardiac cycle number and drug concentration in the left ventricle?

Assume a left ventricle whose contractile characteristics are the same as those of the left ventricle in example 1.1. In this example C_{target} = 0 mg/L.

- Initial drug concentration = C_0 = 100 mg/L.

- The left ventricle contracts, ejecting 67% of the blood and drug present, which means that only 33% of the drug present in the left ventricle remains. At the end of the first subsequent diastole 67% of the left ventricle is filled with blood containing no drug. So;

$$C_1 = 100 \times 0.33 = 33 \text{ mg/L}$$

-    At the end of the next cardiac cycle, 67% of the drug present has again been ejected and replaced with blood containing no drug, reducing the left ventricular drug concentration to 33% of that in the previous cycle. So;

$$C_2 = 100 \times 0.33 \times 0.33 = 100 \times 0.33^2 = 10.89 \text{ mg/L}$$

-    Similarly, for the next diastolic period.

$$C_3 = 100 \times 0.33^2 \times 0.33 = 100 \times 0.33^3 = 3.59 \text{ mg/L}$$

The general equation giving drug concentration in the left ventricle at any cardiac cycle number after drug injection is therefore given by equation 1.2.

$$C_n = 100 \times 0.33^n \qquad (1.2)$$

The same method used in example 1.1 can also be used to show that the reduction of drug concentration from one cardiac cycle to the next is also a constant fraction of the DIFFERENCE between the existing and the target drug concentration.

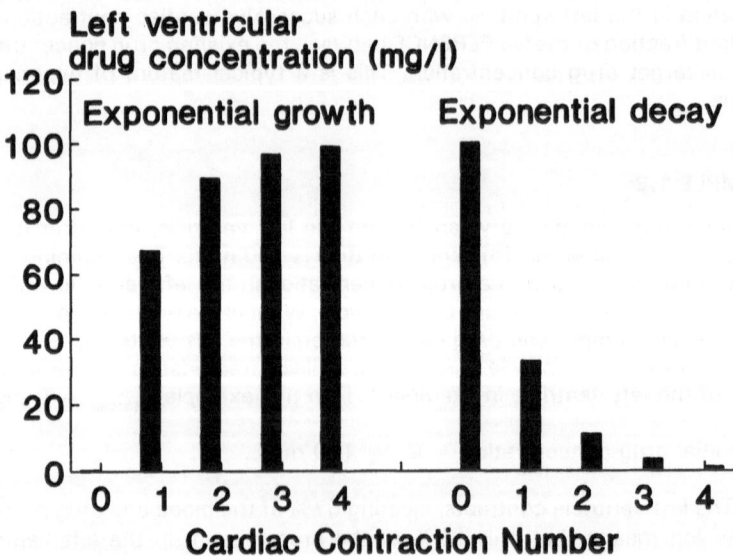

Figure 1.1: This figure shows the exponential growth and decay of the intraventricular drug concentration with successive cardiac contractions as discussed in examples 1.1 and 1.2.

Example 1.1 is an example of a process showing EXPONENTIAL GROWTH, while example 1.2 is a typical example of EXPONENTIAL DECAY. Both examples show that a basic property of an exponentially changing process is that the magnitude of the change that occurs within a given interval is NOT a constant fraction of the difference between the original amount or level of a quantity and the target level. Instead the magnitude of the change is a constant fraction of the difference between the level existing at the start of an interval and the target level or amount.

General form of the exponential equation

Examples 1.1 and 1.2 show the basic form of an exponential equation. This is the same regardless of whether the equation describes exponential decay or growth. The basic equation of an exponential function is shown by equation 1.3. Readers should take careful note that the general form of the exponential equation is the same as that of a "power function". The difference between a power function and an exponential function is that the exponent of a power function is constant and the base is variable, while for an exponential finction, the base is constant and the exponent variable.

$$y = b^x \qquad (1.3)$$

x is the exponent, and this may be any positive or negative real number.
b is the "base" of the exponent. The base of an exponential function is a **constant**.
y is the product of the exponential function.

Exponential functions with the base "e"

While it is true that the base of an exponential function may be any real number, mathematicians usually try to convert all exponential equation bases to the number "e". This is because of the unique properties of this number. Exponential equations using "e" as a base are readily manipulated using the techniques of differential and integral calculus. The number "e" itself is a "transcendental" number just like "π". Like π, "e" also has an infinite number of non-repeating decimal places. The value of "e" accurate to five decimal places is 2.71828. Exponential equations using "e" as a base have the same form as any other exponential equation [see equation 1.4].

$$y = e^x \qquad (1.4)$$

LOGARITHMIC FUNCTIONS

Logarithms are derived from exponential functions and share the same properties. A logarithm may be defined thus: If "y" is the product of the exponential function "b^x", then the exponent "x" is the logarithm of "y" to the base "b". This definition becomes clearer when the general exponential equation, equation 1.3, is compared with this definition.

$$y = b^x \qquad (1.3)$$

The logarithmic form of this exponential equation is;

$$log_b y = x \qquad (1.5)$$

In other words, the base of a logarithm is the same as the base of the corresponding exponential equation. The base of a logarithmic equation can only be a positive real number other than one. This is because the product of one raised to any power is one, and so it is useless to use this as a base for either a logarithmic or exponential function.

The base of a logarithm determines the purposes for which it is used. Two types of logarithms are in common use. These are logarithms to the base "e" or "natural logarithms", and logarithms to the base 10 or "common logarithms".

Logarithms to the base 10 (log, log_{10})

"Common" logarithms are logarithms using 10 as a base. They are usually represented in one of two ways, either by log_{10} or simply by log. This type of logarithm is particularly suited for performing arithmetical calculations and for graphical purposes.

Performing arithmetical calculations

Common logarithms are particularly suited for performing arithmetical calculations involving division, multiplication and exponents.

Graphical purposes

Another use of common logarithms is for graphical purposes. The reason for this lies in the way that common logarithms represent powers of 10. For example:

Exponential form	Logarithmic form
$10 = 10^1$	$log(10) = 1$
$100 = 10^2$	$log(100) = 2$
$1000 = 10^3$	$log(1000) = 3$
$10000 = 10^4$	$log(10000) = 4$

So it is evident that common logarithms can represent powers of ten with integers which can be readily put on a linear scale. Conversion of the scale of one or more axes of a graph to common logarithms is useful in situations where the "x", "y" or both data ranges are large. It is then possible to fit all the data on one graph.

Logarithmic graphical axes are also very useful when representing exponential processes. If the y-axis of the graph of a process undergoing exponential change is converted to common logarithms, the graph is changed from an exponential to a linear graph which is much more easily read [see figure 1.2]. Such a graph is called a semi-logarithmic graph, as only one axis has data in logarithmic form.

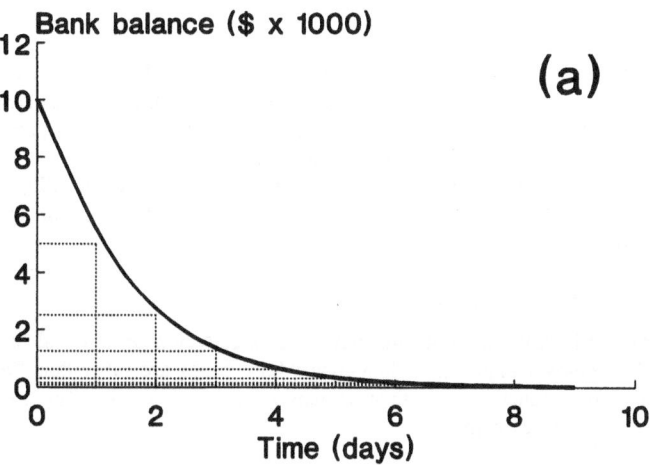

Figure 1.2: A person has a bank account containing $10,000. Each day he removes a sum of money equal to one half of the amount of money remaining in the account on that day. On day one, the balance halves to $5000. On day two it halves to $2500, and on day three it halves yet again, leaving only $1250 in the account. This process continues until the account has been emptied. Figure 1.2a shows this process with two linear axes. Unfortunately it is impossible to use figure 1.2a to accurately read the amount of money remaining in the account after four days. This problem has been solved in figure 1.2b by using a logarithmic y-axis which has made the curve linear, increasing the accuracy and utility of the graph.

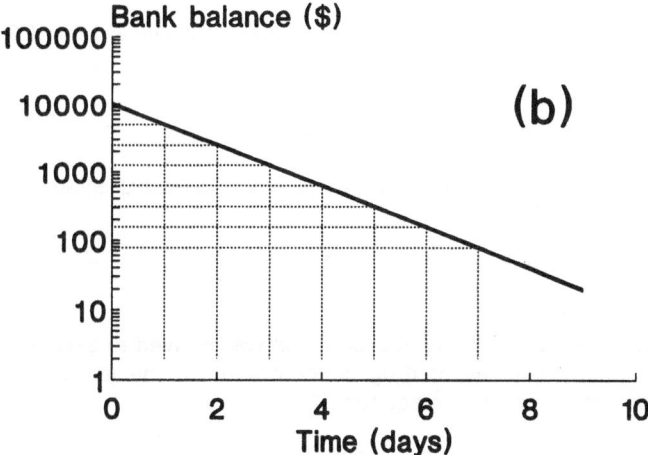

Natural logarithms (ln, or log_e)

Natural logarithms are logarithms to the base "e" (e = 2.71828). They are usually denoted by **ln** or **log_e**. As with exponentials to the base "e", natural logarithms are also easily manipulated using differential and integral calculus. Natural logarithms frequently arise as part of the solutions of the differential equations describing drug kinetics and dynamics.

There are two basic uses of natural logarithms which are worthwhile explaining more extensively in this book. Conversion of exponential bases to exponentials with base "e", and the concept of "half life".

Conversion of exponential bases to "e"

Exponential and logarithmic functions may have bases which are any real number. However it is often useful to convert exponential functions whose bases are other than "e", to functions whose base is "e". These functions may then be manipulated more easily. This may be done using equation 1.7 which is derived below.

Equation 1.6 describes the relationship between an exponential function with a base "b" which can be any number, and an exponential function with base "e".

$$e^{kt} = b^{xt} \tag{1.6}$$

In this equation both exponential terms have a double exponent, in one case "xt", and the other "kt". "x" and "k" are constants, while "t" is a known variable part of the exponent.

From the definition of logarithms [see equation 1.5];

$$\ln(b^{xt}) = kt$$

If "b", "x" and "t" are known then "k" may be calculated with equation 1.7;

$$k = \frac{\ln(b^{xt})}{t} \tag{1.7}$$

The utility of formula 1.7 for conversion of monoexponential equation bases to "e" is illustrated with example 1.3.

EXAMPLE 1.3:

In example 1.2 an exponential equation was derived to describe the time related exponential decay of drug concentration in the left ventricle. The general equation derived was equation 1.2.

$$C_n = 100 \times 0.33^n \tag{1.2}$$

After 3 contractions the ventricular drug concentration is;

$$C_3 = 100 \times 0.33^3$$

These values may be substituted into equation 1.7 to get;

$$k = \frac{\ln(0.33^3)}{3} = -1.108$$

The resulting exponential equation to the base "e" is therefore;

$$C_n = 100 \times e^{-1.108n} \qquad (1.8)$$

The results obtained using this equation are the same as with equation 1.2. This equation is a typical example of a mono-exponential equation to the base "e" describing a process undergoing exponential decay.

Natural logarithms and "Half life"

Figures 1.1 and 1.2a show that it is very difficult to determine the exact point at which an exponentially changing process is complete. However it is useful to have some idea as to when the change that an exponential process undergoes is nearly or totally finished. One measure that is used for this purpose is given by the very definition of an exponential process. The degree of change per unit time is a constant fraction of the difference between the current level or quantity of a variable and the target level of that variable. This statement means that a given percentage change of a quantity or amount takes the same amount of time regardless of the absolute value of that change. So what is required is to select a convenient percentage degree of change. By convention, and also because of computational ease, the time taken for an amount or quantity to double, or be reduced by a half is chosen. This is the **half life** of a process.

A half life may be defined as that time required for the amount or quantity of a parameter undergoing exponential change to double, or be reduced by one half of the difference between the level at the beginning of the half life period and the target level.

The equation defining the half life of an exponential process can be derived using the properties of natural logarithms. Consider equation 1.9. This is a general monoexponential equation whose base is "e" which describes a decay process.

$$C = C_0 . e^{-kt} \qquad (1.9)$$

t is time.
k is a constant.
C_0 is the amount, concentration, or quantity of a parameter at time = 0.
C is the amount, concentration, or quantity of a parameter after time = t has elapsed.

The time taken for C_0 to halve is given by rearranging equation 1.9 so that;

$$\frac{C}{C_0} = \frac{1}{2} = e^{-kt}$$

Using equation 1.5, which is the definition of logarithms, and after rearranging, the final equation defining the "half life" ($t_{1/2}$) is;

$$t_{1/2} = -\frac{\ln(1/2)}{k} = \frac{0.693}{k} \tag{1.10}$$

The half life principle can be applied to drug kinetics and dynamics too. The half life gives a measure of how long it takes for a monoexponential process to be nearly complete. Table 1.1 shows that a monoexponential process is about 90% complete after a time equivalent to 3-4 times the $t_{1/2}$ has elapsed. This is an important relationship and is used repeatedly throughout this book.

Table 1.1.

Relationship between the multiple of the half life of a substance and the amount or concentration of that substance present during situations where MONOEXPONENTIAL growth or decay occur.

Multiple of the half life	GROWTH Amount of a substance as % of TARGET amount (original amount = 0 and target = 100)	DECAY Amount of a substance as % of ORIGINAL amount (original amount = 100 and target = 0)
0	0	100
1	50	50
2	75	25
3	87.5	12.5
4	93.75	6.25
5	96.875	3.125

EXAMPLE 1.4:

What is the half life of the exponential process described by equation 1.8;

$$C_n = 100 \times e^{-1.108n} \qquad (1.8)$$

This is the exponential equation to the base "e" describing the time related decrease of drug concentration in the left ventricle at any cardiac conctraction cycle number [see example 1.2]. Use equation 1.10 to calculate the half life of the drug in the left ventricle.

$$t_{1/2} = \frac{0.693}{k} = \frac{0.693}{1.108} = 0.625 \text{ contractions.}$$

This means that the amount of drug in the left ventricle halves with each 0.625 contraction.

BASIC ELEMENTS OF KINETIC MODELLING

Regardless of their nature, all pharmacokinetic, and some pharmacodynamic models, are based on one basic concept, the "compartment". A pharmacokinetic or pharmacodynamic compartment may be defined as a physical, anatomical or functional volume where drug enters and leaves, and throughout which the drug is evenly distributed. Understanding of the consequences of this concept is central to any deeper understanding of drug kinetics and dynamics. Examples of different sorts of pharmacokinetic compartments are given below.

- Consider a tank of water which is continuously stirred. Water flows through a pipe into this tank at a fixed rate. The water flows out of the tank through another pipe at the same rate. Mixing of any substance entering the tank in the water flowing into the tank, or added to the water in the tank is rapid and complete. The tank is an example of a physically well defined compartment.

- Another example is the right ventricle. Blood flow into, and out of the right ventricle is equal to the cardiac output. The volume of the ventricle changes, but the end-diastolic and end-systolic volumes are otherwise anatomically well defined. Intravenously injected drugs enter the right ventricle, are fully distributed throughout the ventricular volume by the turbulent movement of blood within it, and are then pumped into the pulmonary circulation. So the situation is the same as in the mechanical example above. This is also an example of a physically or anatomically well defined compartment.

- In most situations occurring in humans and animals, neither the anatomical volumes nor the blood flows of the compartments in which an administered drug distribute are known. Despite this, the distribution of that drug can be described quite accurately using the drug compartment concept. So while the drug containing compartments do not actually exist as physical or anatomical entities, they do function as compartments. Such compartments are examples of "functional" compartments.

The mathematical treatment of a compartment is the same regardless of whether the volume is well defined by anatomical or physical bounds, or is a functional compartment whose volume is not so easily defined.

This section will now discuss the basic principles of the mathematical treatment of pharmacokinetic compartments. These principles are used in nearly all chapters of this book. Because of this the reader is encouraged to persevere and read this section. While the application of the equations may not be immediately apparent, their practical solutions and uses are explained fully in the latter part of this section.

Calculation of drug concentration

Prior to any further discussion on particular pharmacokinetic models, it is well worth reviewing the basic equation used to calculate all drug concentrations. Drug concentration in any pharmacokinetic compartment, regardless of whether the volume of the compartment is anatomically well defined, or whether it is only functional, is given by the same equation. This is equation 1.11. It is fundamental to all pharmacokinetic models.

$$\text{Concentration} = C = \frac{\text{Amount}}{\text{Volume}} = \frac{\text{Dose}}{V} \tag{1.11}$$

Figure 1.3: This figure shows a single physically or anatomically well defined compartment of volume "V". Fluid flows into, and out of this compartment at the same rate "F". Drug is dissolved in the incoming fluid with concentration equal to "C_{in}".

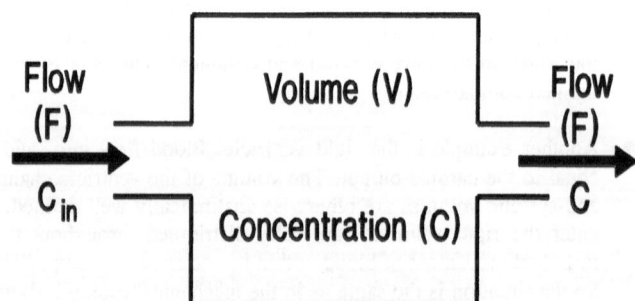

A single compartment where INFLOW = OUTFLOW

The simplest type of compartment is one where fluid flows into the compartment at the same rate as it flows out. This is depicted in figure 1.3. Mixing of the fluid within the compartment is rapid and complete, so the concentration of any drug is the same throughout the compartment. It is possible by using some basic principles to derive equations describing the rate of change of drug concentration with time for any drug within the compartment for two situations commonly encountered in drug kinetics and clinical practice.

- The situation where a drug is injected into the compartment in a single rapid dose. A clinical equivalent of this is a rapid intra-atrial or intravenous injection of a drug dose, [see equation 1.16].

- A continuous flow of drug containing fluid enters the compartment. The clinical equivalent of this is a continuous intravenous infusion of a drug, [see equation 1.15].

The single compartment model that will now be developed to describe these two situations uses the following notation.

δ is a conventional symbol meaning a very small change of a given value or parameter.
M is the amount or dose of drug.
F is the flow rate of the fluid into and out of the compartment.
V is the volume of the compartment.
C_{in} is the concentration of the drug in the fluid flowing into the compartment.
C is the concentration of the drug inside the compartment. Because mixing within the compartment is so rapid and complete, it is also the concentration of that drug in the fluid flowing out of the compartment.
t is time.

Drug dissolved in incoming fluid

Figure 1.3 depicts a situation where the fluid entering a single compartment contains a drug at a concentration given by C_{in}. The rate of fluid flow out of the compartment is the same as the rate of fluid flow into the compartment. Change in the amount of drug (δM) within the compartment in a small time interval δt is the difference between the amount of drug entering and the amount of drug leaving the compartment in that time interval δt.

$$\delta M = C_{in}.F.\delta t - C.F.\delta t \qquad (1.12)$$

Divide both sides of the equation by the volume of the compartment to get an expression for the change of concentration in the time interval δt.

$$\frac{\delta M}{V} = \delta C = \frac{F.\delta t}{V} (C_{in} - C)$$ (1.13)

Divide both sides by δt to get the rate of change of concentration.

$$\frac{\delta C}{\delta t} = \frac{F}{V} (C_{in} - C)$$ (1.14)

If the interval "δ" is made infinitesimally small, the same conditions apply, and the more usual symbol "d" from differential calculus can be used. Equation 1.14 may then be rewritten as equation 1.15.

$$\frac{dC}{dt} = \frac{F}{V} (C_{in} - C)$$ (1.15)

The reader should not take fright at the use of this terminology. All that dC/dt stands for is the rate of change of concentration, e.g. grams/100 mls/second, picomoles/cubic meter/day, or milligrams/liter/minute etc.

Equation 1.15 does show one very interesting fact. The ratio F/V is constant for a given flow and compartment volume. Rate of change of drug concentration within a compartment is therefore purely a function of the difference between C_{in} and C multiplied by the constant F/V. Restated, this means that the rate of change of concentration within the compartment is a constant fraction of the difference between the target concentration and the present concentration. That is, the change of concentration with time is an exponential process.

Single dose of drug injected into one compartment

Here the total amount of the drug is injected rapidly into a single drug containing compartment. The situation is identical to that where the drug continuously enters the compartment dissolved in the incoming fluid, except that the incoming fluid contains no drug. Thus $C_{in} = 0$, and equation 1.15 reduces to equation 1.16.

$$\frac{dC}{dt} = - C \frac{F}{V}$$ (1.16)

Rate constants

The ratio F/V used in the specific model above is an example of what is called a rate constant. A rate constant is usually given the symbol "k", and has the unit **time**$^{-1}$. This somewhat unusual unit may be confirmed by what is called "dimensional analysis". Dimensional analysis is a method by which the various dimensions of each variable in an equation are set out in the form of the equation, and those which are equivalent but opposite in sign cancelled out. The remaining dimensions are those of the product of the equation.

For example, for the rate constant F/V, this is done as follows;

$$\frac{F}{V} = \frac{\cancel{volume}}{time} \times \frac{1}{\cancel{volume}} = \frac{1}{time} = time^{-1}$$

The rate constant is the fractional volume of drug containing fluid entering or leaving a pharmacokinetic compartment per unit time. This made more obvious with an example.

EXAMPLE 1.5:

Consider the right ventricle. Assume that at the end of diastole it contains blood in which a drug is dissolved. The right ventricle never completely empties during systole, in fact only 0.5 or 50% of the end-diastolic-volume is ejected as the stroke volume. This means that with each contraction 50% of the drug contained within the right ventricle is ejected, and so 50% of the drug remains.

Assume that no more drug enters the right ventricle. So after one contraction only 50% of the original amount of drug present at the end of the preceding diastole remains. If no more drug enters during the next diastole, then this remaining drug mixes with, and is diluted by incoming blood during the next diastolic period. During the next systole, 50% of the remaining drug is ejected, and the whole process repeats itself.

In this example the rate constant is the "ejection fraction", which is the fractional emptying of the right ventricle during systole, (ejection fraction = stroke volume / end diastolic volume). It is also apparent that the rate constant says nothing about how much drug is ejected in a given time interval, or in this case per contraction, but only says what fraction of the volume of the drug containing fluid present in the compartment is ejected in that time interval.

A general 1-compartment equation

The above discussion has dealt with a very specific 1-compartment model, one where the rate of fluid flow into a compartment equals the rate at which it flows out. This is not always encountered in practice. So the 1-compartment model concept will now be generalized to describe situations where the rate of flow into a compartment does not necessarily equal the rate of flow out of that compartment, [see figure 1.4].

The equation for a generally applicable 1-compartment drug model is given by equation 1.17.

Figure 1.4: A generalized 1-compartment model. The rate constant of drug entry is denoted by "k_{in}" and that for drug exit by "k_{out}".

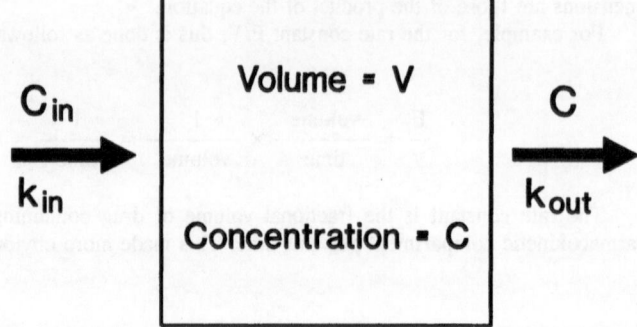

$$\frac{dC}{dt} = C_{in}.k_{in} - C.k_{out} \tag{1.17}$$

C_{in} is the concentration of drug in the incoming fluid.
C is the concentration of drug in the fluid flowing out of the compartment, and at the same time the concentration of drug in the fluid inside the compartment.
k_{in} is the fractional rate constant for drug entry into the compartment.
k_{out} is the fractional rate constant for drug exit from the compartment.

This model may be applied to any 1-compartment drug model where drug is either injected directly into the compartment, or is dissolved in the incoming fluid.

Multiple compartment models

The same methods used for the 1-compartment model may also be used for models containing more than one compartment. A multiple or multi-compartment model may be considered as consisting of several single compartments. As with the 1-compartment model, drug enters and leaves each compartment. All that is necessary to derive equations describing the rate of change of drug concentration in any given compartment, is to derive an equation for each compartment separately.

This principle will now be illustrated by being applied to two variations of a 2-compartment model. These models are shown in figures 1.5a and 1.5b.

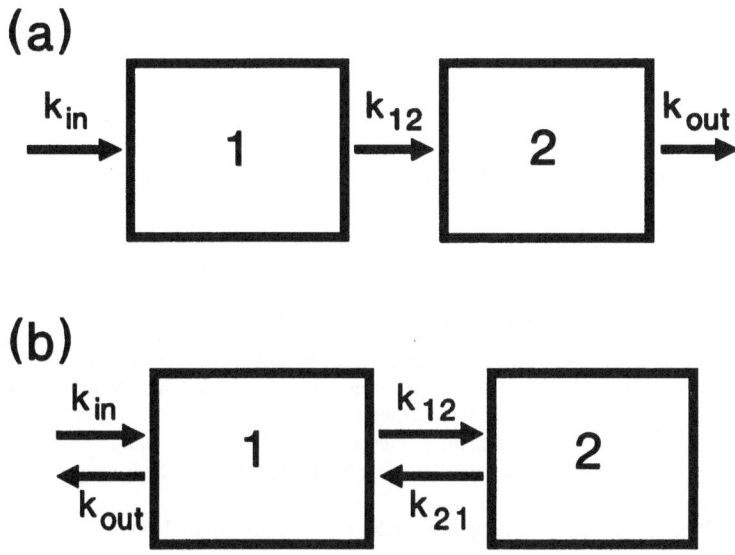

Figure 1.5: Figure 1.5a and figure 1.5b show two variations of a 2-compartment model. The volume of, and drug concentration within, compartment number-1 are termed "V_1" and "C_1" respectively, and for compartment number-2 these terms are "V_2" and "C_2". Drug is exchanged between the two compartments, or flows from compartment-1 to compartment-2. The rate constants are given a subscript, the first number of which is the compartment of origin, while the second number is the compartment to which the drug flows.

Figure 1.5a: Compartment-1 feeds compartment-2

Consider the 2-compartment model to be made up of two separate single compartments, each compartment with its own rate of input and output of the drug under consideration. Application of the basic principles discussed for a 1-compartment model enables two equations to be derived. One equation gives the rate of change of drug concentration in compartment-1 and the other in compartment-2.

For compartment-1;

$$\frac{dC_1}{dt} = C_{in}.k_{in} - C_1.k_{12} \tag{1.18}$$

Compartment-2 is fed by compartment-1, and it is from compartment-2 that the drug leaves the 2-compartment system. So the equation for compartment-2 is;

$$\frac{dC_2}{dt} = C_1.k_{12} - C_2.k_{out} \tag{1.19}$$

C_1, C_2, C_{in} are drug concentrations in compartments 1, 2 and in the fluid entering compartment-1 respectively.
k_{in}, k_{12}, k_{out} are rate constants.

Figure 1.5b: Drug is exchanged between two compartments

The 2-compartment model depicted in figure 1.5b differs from that in figure 1.5a in that drug input into and output from the 2-compartment system occurs only through compartment-1. In this system, the only way that drug enters compartment-2 is from compartment-1, and the only way it leaves compartment-2 is into compartment-1. Despite these differences, the approach is the same. Consider each compartment as a separate single compartment into which drug enters and from which it leaves.

The resulting equations describing the model depicted in figure 1.5b are:

$$\frac{dC_1}{dt} = C_{in}.k_{in} + C_2.k_{21} - C_1.k_{12} - C_1.k_{out} \tag{1.20}$$

$$\frac{dC_2}{dt} = C_1.k_{12} - C_2.k_{21} \tag{1.21}$$

The 2-compartment model described by figure 1.5b is important. It is used in many studies of the kinetics of anesthetic drugs, and is also used extensively throughout this book too. Further discussion of the properties of this model is to be found in chapter 2.

Solution of equations in this section

It is all very interesting to be able to calculate the rate of change of concentration of a drug in any given drug containing compartment, but a practical person would rather know the drug concentration. Drug effect is nearly always related to the concentration of a drug, rather than the rate of change of drug concentration.

All the equations giving the rate of change of drug concentration derived in this section are of the type called differential equations. Regrettably for the mathematically less gifted, the derivation of exact solutions of these differential equations is not possible without knowledge of, and ability to use calculus. In the case of multi-compartment model equations where there is a whole series of interrelated equations, a knowledge of advanced calculus is necessary.

Fortunately with the current ready availability of powerful and cheap microcomputers, a knowledge of advanced calculus is not necessary in order to use the equations derived in this section. It is possible to use a microcomputer to solve these differential equations, and so calculate the drug concentrations at any time in each compartment of a model. The simplest technique available to do this is Euler's method. There are other techniques, but Euler's method will be the only one discussed here as it is sufficient for the purposes of most pharmacokinetic analyses. The interested reader can read about the many other numerical, (computer), methods of solving differential equations in any standard work on numerical analysis.

Euler's method

Here we will only consider the specific application of Euler's method to solving pharmacokinetic equations of the type developed for pharmacokinetic compartments in this chapter. Consider a differential equation of the type shown as equation 1.22. This equation gives the rate of change of concentration of a drug as being equal to "A", which may be a constant or an equation.

$$\frac{dC}{dt} = A \qquad (1.22)$$

It is desired to solve this equation for "C" so that the concentration can be calculated at a given time. The procedure to be followed is:

1. Let "dt" be a small but significant time interval.

2. If "dt" is known then the magnitude of the change "dC" has undergone in that time interval can be calculated by rearranging equation 1.22 to equation 1.23:

$$dC = A.dt \qquad (1.23)$$

3. The new concentration (C_{new}) is then simply calculated by adding "dC" to the previous drug concentration (C_{old}).

$$C_{new} = C_{old} + dC \qquad (1.24)$$

which may also be expressed as equation 1.25.

$$C_{new} = C_{old} + A.dt \qquad (1.25)$$

4. Steps 2 and 3 are repeated indefinitely, or for as long as desired. When these steps are repeated, the "C_{new}" calculated in the previous cycle becomes the "C_{old}" for the new cycle.

5. The elapsed time is given by the number of times steps 2 and 3 have been repeated, multiplied by "dt".

Figure 1.6: The 1-com-
partment model used in
example 1.6.

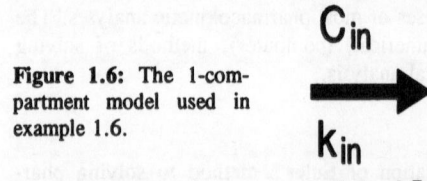
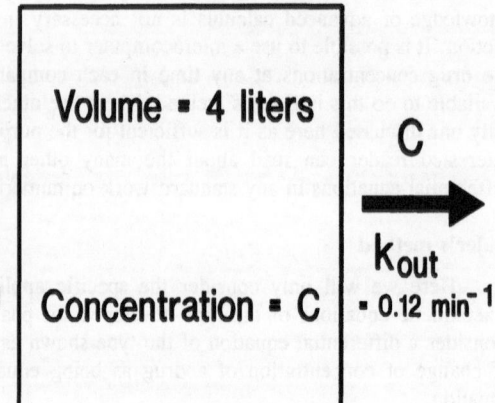

C_{in}

k_{in}

$= 0.3 \text{ min}^{-1}$

Volume = 4 liters

Concentration = C

C

k_{out}

$= 0.12 \text{ min}^{-1}$

EXAMPLE 1.6:

Consider a single compartment into which a drug is infused. The volume of this compartment is not necessarily anatomically well defined. Incoming drug concentration $= C_{in} = 100$ mg/L, $k_{in} = 0.3$ min^{-1}, and $k_{out} = 0.12$ min^{-1} [see figure 1.6].

Use Euler's method to calculate the drug concentration in the compartment after 0.4 minutes when the initial drug concentration $= C_{old} = 0$ mg/L.

The equation describing the rate of change of drug concentration in this single compartment with time is given by;

$$\frac{dC}{dt} = C_{in}.k_{in} - C.k_{out} = 0.3C_{in} - 0.12C$$

This may be substituted into equation 1.25 to get;

$$C_{new} = C_{old} + dt(0.3C_{in} - 0.12C_{old})$$

Let dt = 0.1 minute, and using the above equation, the drug concentrations within the compartment at various times can be calculated as follows.

At time = 0 minutes;
C_{old} = 0 mg/L.

At time = 0.1 minutes;
C_{new} = 0 + 0.1(0.3 x 100 - 0.12 x 0) = 3 mg/L

At time = 0.2 minutes;
C_{new} = 3 + 0.1(0.3 x 100 - 0.12 x 3) = 5.964 mg/L

At time = 0.3 minutes;
C_{new} = 5.964 + 0.1(0.3 x 100 - 0.12 x 5.964) = 8.892 mg/L

At time = 0.4 minutes;
C_{new} = 8.892 + 0.1(0.3 x 100 - 0.12 x 8.892) = 11.79 mg/L

Implementation of Euler's method on a microcomputer

It is evident from example 1.6 that manual execution of the calculations required when using Euler's method for solving differential equations can be tedious and time consuming. The microcomputer is an exceptionally capable aid with this type of equation, being rapid, tireless, and not so prone to make arithmetical errors as a human. There are two ways this method may actually be implemented on a microcomputer.

- A program may be written in a programming language familiar to the user, and this program performs the necessary calculations providing output in the form of a table, a graph or both.

- A second much simpler method is to use a type of program called a "spreadsheet". Spreadsheet programs are widely available for a large number of different computer systems. Modern versions implement a large range of mathematical functions, as well as providing tabular and graphical output of calculations. Their main advantage is that no knowledge of computer programming languages is required on the part of the user.

Limitations of Euler's method

Euler's method is simple, and is usually more than sufficient for most purposes in solving equations of multi-compartment models, but the reader should be aware that there is a major problem with its use. The Euler method is what is called a "one-step" method for solving differential equations. If the interval chosen is too large, ("dt" in the examples above), the results of the calculations are wildly inaccurate. Accuracy of results obtained with Euler's method increase with smaller time intervals. The best interval to use is usually determined empirically by calculations performed with different time intervals. If the results with different intervals are significantly different, then the procedure should be repeated with smaller intervals until the differences between results obtained with different and smaller intervals are minimal.

For most purposes in pharmacokinetics it is sufficient to let the interval, usually a time interval "dt", be $1/10^{th}$ of the unit of time under consideration. For example if the time span under consideration is best measured in seconds, let dt = 0.1 second, and if minutes are used let dt = 0.1 minute, etc.

Chapter 2

Physiological Aspects of Drug Kinetics and Dynamics

Before discussing the pharmacokinetic and pharmacodynamic models in current use, it is well worth discussing their physiological basis. This has several advantages.

- A physiological approach to drug kinetics describes the actual distribution and elimination of drugs.

- Anesthesiologists usually view and solve most problems in physiological terms. Therefore such an approach is one which simplifies learning drug kinetics and dynamics by using familiar concepts.

- An appreciation of the physiological basis of the currently used kinetic and dynamic models makes it easier to predict changes resulting from any disturbance of normal physiology.

- An appreciation of the physiological basis of drug distribution and elimination also shows some of the limitations of current pharmacokinetic models.

CIRCULATION TIME

The first question a pragmatic physician asks himself after injecting a drug intravenously is; "How soon after administration will the drug arrive at the organs on which it exerts its effect?" This is a question which can be answered with knowledge of the relevant circulation times. A circulation time is simply the time taken for a drug injected into the vascular system at one point to APPEAR at another point in the vascular system. It should be noted that the term "appear" does not mean peak concentration. Table 2.1 lists a variety of circulation times between various points in the body. These circulation times show that it takes a short but finite time for any intravenously or intra-arterially administered drug to arrive anywhere in the body.

Circulation time is a parameter that was frequently used in the past as a measure of cardiac output. The most frequently used circulation time was the time taken for a substance to arrive at the tongue after injection into a forearm vein, the arm-to-tongue circulation time. Substances such as quinine, calcium gluconate, or saccharine were used as their arrival in the tongue is signaled by the appropriate taste. Fluorescein was another commonly used marker substance, the arrival of which at any point is easily observed with an ultraviolet lamp.

Table 2.1.
Circulation times measured in resting healthy adult humans between various points in the vascular system [1].

Vascular circuit	Circulation time (seconds)
Arm vein to right atrium	6.4-7.3
Arm vein to lung	6-8
Arm vein to left ventricle	5-8
Arm vein to tongue	12-15
Arm vein to brain	13-20
Arm vein to arm	12-30
Arm vein to foot	20-37
Foot vein to lung	32
Foot vein to tongue	37-47
Right ventricle to left ventricle	1.7
Right heart to radial artery	10.7
Right heart to ear	8

The time required for a substance injected at one point in the vascular system to appear at another point is related to both the blood flow and the volume of blood in the vascular system between those two points [see figure 2.1]. An injected substance must fill the vascular volume between the points of injection and sampling before it can appear at the sampling point. So the circulation time is related to, but not necessarily equal to, the blood volume divided by the blood flow between the injection and sampling points according to equation 2.1.

$$\text{Circulation time } \alpha \ \frac{\text{Volume}}{\text{Flow}} \tag{2.1}$$

Volume is the volume of blood vessels, and hence blood volume, through which a substance must flow after being injected at one point in the circu/lation, and being detected at another point. **Flow** is the blood flow between the injection and sampling points.

Equation 2.1 shows that it will take less time for any drug to arrive at any point in the body after intravascular injection in conditions where cardiac output is increased, and vice versa. Clinical investigation and practice both confirm this relationship [1]. For example, most anesthetists know from experience that it takes a longer time for drugs such as intravenous induction agents to act after intravenous injection in elderly persons with cardiac disease than in healthy young persons.

Figure 2.1: A drug will not appear at a more distal sampling point until the intervening blood volume is first filled by blood containing that drug.

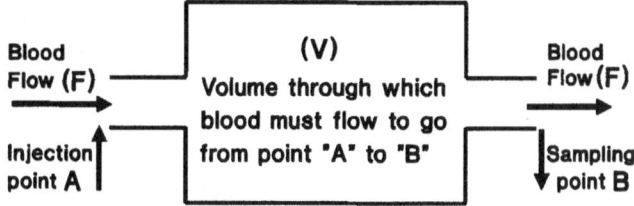

TRANSFER OF DRUG FROM BLOOD TO TISSUE

Once a drug has arrived at tissues in which it is active, it must move out of the blood vessels if it is to affect the cells of those tissues. A person does not experience pain relief from opiates, fall asleep because of the administration of hypnotic drugs, nor become paralyzed due to muscle relaxants because blood cells experience pain relief, fall asleep, or become paralyzed. These drugs all act by affecting the functioning of extravascular cells. Movement of drugs out of capillaries can be quite rapid as is well shown by the rapidity with which some drugs act.
Thiopental induces sleep within 15-25 seconds in the average adult after rapid intravenous injection of 4-6 mg/kg into a forearm or cubital vein. Table 2.1 shows that thiopental simply does not arrive in the brain until 13-20 seconds have passed after intravenous injection. After thiopental arrives in the brain, cerebral tissue concentrations of thiopental evidently increase very rapidly in about 2-12 seconds to a concentration sufficient to induce sleep.

- A similar situation occurs with succinylcholine after rapid injection of 1 mg/kg into a forearm or cubital fossa vein. Muscle paralysis is induced in all muscles in less than 45 seconds. Table 2.1 shows that it will take the drug at most about 12-15 seconds to reach the head, 12-30 seconds to reach the arms, and 20-37 seconds to reach the foot. Again, the drug has very little time in which to leave the blood vessels and induce muscle relaxation. A small note can be added here, the sequence of circulation times listed here nicely shows what experienced anesthesiologists have always noted for many years. Muscle fasciculations induced by succinylcholine always begin in the head and neck, subsequently the arms and lastly the legs and feet.

How is it possible for drugs to move out of capillaries and act so rapidly? The explanation of this requires some discussion of the processes by which drugs leave the blood to enter extravascular tissues. There are three processes by which this occurs, active transport, bulk flow and diffusion.

Active transport

Active transport of drugs from the blood vessels into the tissues where they are active or distributed does not occur to any significant degree with any of the drugs used in anesthetic practice.

Bulk flow

Drugs cannot diffuse out of veins and arteries. The only blood vessels whose walls are permeable to drugs are venules and capillaries. Capillaries have pores whose sizes vary from one capillary bed to the other. In general, capillary pore diameters range from 3 to 4.5 nanometers [2,3]. Such pores are usually intercellular crevices, although pores have actually been observed to pass directly through some endothelial cells. A diameter of 3-4.5 nanometers means that these pores are too small to permit the passage of blood cells. This pore size is also small enough to restrict the movement of larger molecules contained in plasma. For example, albumin has a molecular weight of 66,271 g/mole and a molecular diameter of 3.6 nanometers. Capillary endothelium is relatively impermeable to albumin, as a molecule whose diameter is nearly the same as that of the capillary pores can only pass through with difficulty [2,3]. Studies of the intravascular to intercellular fluid concentration ratios of protein molecules confirm this. In addition, it has also been shown that capillary endothelium is relatively permeable to molecules whose molecular weight is less than 10,000 g/mole, while being relatively impermeable to molecules whose molecular weights are greater than 60,000 g/mole [4]. Appendix-B shows that the molecular weights of all drugs used in anesthetic practice are below 1000 g/mole. So anesthetic drugs pass relatively easily through capillary endothelial pores.

All blood vessels are collapsible tubes held open because the pressure of the blood inside them is greater than the pressure exerted on them by the tissues in which they are embedded. If this were not the case, no capillary or venous blood flow would be possible. A good illustration of this principle is the cerebral circulation after massive head trauma. If the intracranial pressure rises high enough, the cerebral circulation ceases because the intravascular pressures are no longer sufficient to keep the cerebral blood vessels patent. This can be demonstrated angiographically in those persons unfortunate enough to have sustained such massive injury.

So capillary blood pressure is higher than the pressure in the surrounding tissues, and the capillaries have pores. This means that capillary blood pressure will force fluid through capillary endothelial pores out of the capillaries into the interstitium. Because of the small sizes of the pores, this fluid is a relatively protein free ultrafiltrate. This process is called "bulk flow". The molecular weights of anesthetic drugs are all below 1000 g/mole, and so these can also move into the pericapillary interstitium by this process.

However, bulk flow is only one of the processes, and certainly not the principal process by which drugs leave capillaries to enter the interstitium. Both experiment and calculation have shown that bulk flow of small molecules is relatively slow in comparison to the rate with which these same molecules can diffuse into the interstitium [2,3].

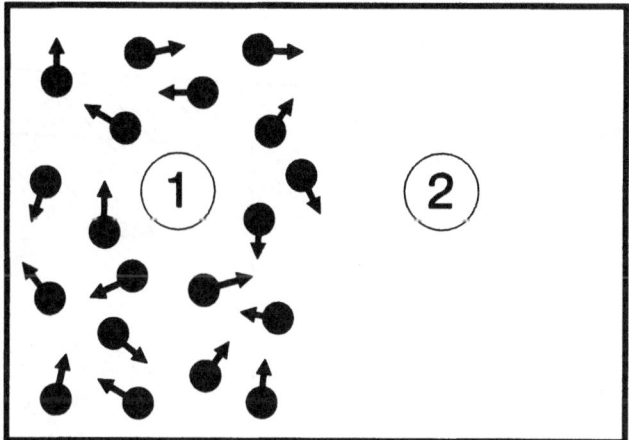

Figure 2.2: This is an imaginary model of a long container filled with a fluid. A substance is dissolved in the fluid in side "1" of the container. Random movement of the solute molecules, (represented by black spots), in side "1" ensures that the solute molecules initially present only in side "1" are eventually present in side "2" too.

Diffusion

Diffusion is the main process by which anesthetic and other drugs move out of capillaries into pericapillary tissues. So it is worthwhile discussing this process in some detail.

The process of diffusion

All molecules in a liquid or gas whose temperature is greater than absolute zero, (= -273° Celsius), are in a state of continuous movement simply by virtue of their thermal kinetic energy. Such molecular movement can be seen with a high powered microscope which is used to view the random movement of extremely fine carbon grains suspended in water. The carbon grains move due to their own thermally induced random movement, and collisions with water molecules also causes them to move. Such thermally caused random molecular movement is called "Brownian movement".

The way in which thermally induced random molecular movement can cause movement of a substance from one place to another may be visualized by imagining a long container in which there is a solute containing fluid. Initially the solute is present in only one end of the container. Random movement of the solute molecules means that at any one time, one half of the solute molecules at a given point in the solution move into fluid in which the solute molecule concentration is lower, and the other half move into regions where it is the same or higher. The result of this is a net movement of molecules from a regions where their concentration is higher to a regions where it is lower. This random dispersal of molecules is called diffusion.

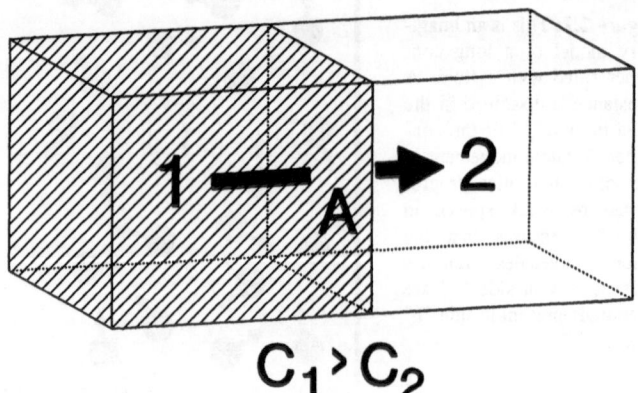

Figure 2.3: Consider a long container containing a fluid. In side "1" of the container a solute is present which is initially not present in side "2". The concentration of the solute is obviously greater in side "1" than in side "2". The area across which the solute molecules can diffuse from side "1" to side "2" is given by "A", in this case the cross sectional area of the container.

The diffusion equation

The basic equation describing the diffusion process was first derived by Fick in 1855. It is often expressed in the form shown by equation 2.2.

$$\frac{dM}{dt} = DA\frac{dC}{dx} \qquad (2.2)$$

A is the area across which diffusion occurs
D is a diffusion constant which is specific for a given solvent and solute.
dM/dt is the is the amount of solute diffusing across area A per unit time.
dC/dx is the change of solute concentration per unit distance.

Figures 2.2 and 2.3 reveal some insights into the most important elements of this equation. The amount of solute (**dM**) that diffuses from section "1" of the long container into section "2" per unit time (**dt**) is related to several parameters.

- **dM/dt** is directly proportional to the area "A" of a membrane, or an interface separating the solvent containing from the non-solvent containing fluid.

- **dM/dt** is also directly proportional to the solute concentration difference (**dC**) per unit distance (**dx**). The greater the concentration difference between any two points, the greater the rate of diffusion and vice versa.

The rate of diffusion, dM/dt in equation 2.2, is directly proportional to the concentration difference between any two points multiplied by the constant "DA". So the Fick diffusion equation also shows that diffusion is an exponential process [see chapter 1 for a more extensive discussion of exponentials]. Regrettably the actual application of such a differential equation in two variables does require a rather good knowledge of calculus. Fortunately solutions of this equation have been worked out for some specific situations. One such solution will be demonstrated as it shows some important properties of the diffusion equation.

Diffusion of drugs out of capillaries, and the "tissue cylinder" model

One of the currently most popular models of capillary-tissue drug exchange is that of a central capillary surrounded by a cylinder of pericapillary tissue [5, and see figure 2.4]. Rate of drug exit from the capillary and entry into the pericapillary tissue cylinder is determined by a number of factors.

- Capillary diameter and endothelial thickness. The average capillary diameter in most tissues is about 6 microns, while capillary endothelium is about 0.3 microns thick.

- Capillary endothelial pore size and density. The larger the pores, and the more of them there are, the more drug that can diffuse out in any given time.

- Drug molecular weight. This determines molecular diameter. Smaller molecules move faster.

- Fat solubility and degree of ionization of the drugs.

- Diameter of the tissue cylinder. The thicker the cuff of tissue surrounding a capillary, the longer it takes a drug to reach the outermost cells. This varies from one organ to the other. In the myocardium and renal cortex tissue cylinder radius is only about 8 microns thick, while in adipose tissue and cerebral white matter an average tissue cylinder is about 34 microns thick [reference 1, page 34].

Equation 2.3 is based on this homogeneous pericapillary tissue cylinder model and shows the change with time of the extravascular drug concentration for a given intracapillary concentration of that same drug [see equations 17 and 18 in reference 2].

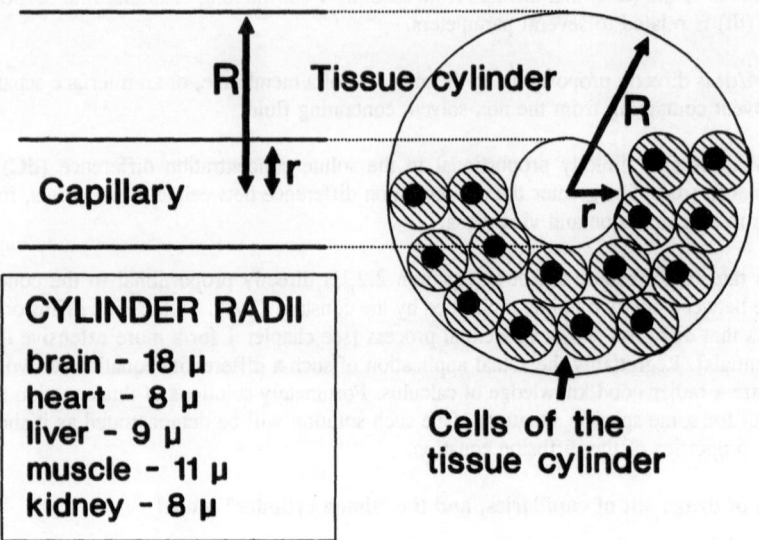

CYLINDER RADII

brain - 18 μ
heart - 8 μ
liver - 9 μ
muscle - 11 μ
kidney - 8 μ

Cells of the tissue cylinder

Figure 2.4: Basic elements of a simple 2-compartment capillary-tissue cylinder model. "R" is the tissue cylinder radius, and "r" the capillary radius.

$$C_e = C_i \cdot \exp\left[t \cdot D \cdot \frac{A}{\delta x} \cdot \frac{(R^2 + r^2)}{R^2 \cdot r^2} \right] \qquad (2.3)$$

C_i and C_e are respectively the intracapillary and the extravascular pericapillary concentrations of a substance or drug.
$A/\delta x$ is the apparent area available for diffusion of a particular molecule per unit path length through the capillary endothelium. This is different for different molecules.
D is the free diffusion coefficient for the specific molecule under consideration.
r is the capillary radius.
R is the tissue cylinder radius.
t is time.

EXAMPLE 2.1:

Consider the diffusion of sucrose out of the capillaries of a cat hind leg. Sucrose is very fat-insoluble with an oil/water partition coefficient of <0.00001, and a molecular weight of 342 g/mole. This molecular weight is of the same order of magnitude as that of many anesthetic drugs [see appendix-B]. The free diffusion coefficient of sucrose in water at 37^OC = 0.75×10^{-5} $cm^2.s^{-1}$. In the normothermic perfused cat hind-leg, for which data are available, A/δx = 0.58×10^{-3} cm/gm muscle tissue [2]. Let the tissue cylinder radius = R = 10 microns = 10^{-3} cm, a figure appropriate for brain and muscle tissue; and capillary radius = r = 3 microns = 3×10^{-4} cm.

Use equation 2.3 and apply the same principles as used in chapter 1 to derive the half-life of a substance or drug. When this is done, it is found that the time required for the tissue cylinder sucrose concentration to be 90% of that in the capillary is 2.38 seconds! This is a very short time indeed. It is evident from this that diffusion is a process by which molecules can rapidly move such small distances.

The above calculation and model are interesting in that they show the basic form of the relevant equations, their exponential nature, and the speed with which drugs can diffuse out of capillaries. However this model does not accurately represent the actual anatomical and physiological situation.

Actual anatomy of tissue cylinders and drug diffusion

The idea of a tissue cylinder is functionally correct, but the tissues within such a cylinder are not homogeneous. Instead a tissue cylinder is made up of cells, in between which is water, connective tissue fibers, and mucopolysaccharide ground substance. This situation is represented somewhat simplistically in the lower half of figure 2.4. Such an anatomy has profound consequences.

Fat-insoluble drugs

Consider the situation of relatively fat-insoluble drugs. These drugs are relatively insoluble in cell membranes. So capillary endothelial cells, and cells in the pericapillary tissues present a barrier to movement of fat-insoluble drugs. This means that relatively fat-insoluble drugs can only leave the capillaries to enter the pericapillary interstitium by movement through capillary pores [2,3]. Membranes of cells within the tissue cylinders also present a barrier to the movement of relatively fat-insoluble drugs, restricting their movement in the tissue cylinder to the spaces between the cells. Such restriction of the movement of fat-insoluble molecules to within the intercellular spaces has been demonstrated using dyes [ref. 33, pages 978-979]. Mucopolysaccharide ground substance and connective tissue fibers in the intercellular spaces further restrict movement of drugs.

Fat-soluble drugs

Fat-soluble drugs are readily soluble in cell membranes. The speed with which fat-soluble drugs can pass through capillary endothelium is very much greater than that possible for fat-insoluble drugs of comparable molecular size and weight. Fat-soluble drugs not only diffuse through the capillary endothelial pores, but can also diffuse through the capillary endothelial cells themselves [3,6]. This same consideration also applies to the cells of the pericapillary tissue cylinder. Movement of fat-soluble drugs is not restricted by cell membranes, and so they are free to diffuse from one area to another through the cells as well as the intercellular spaces.

Speed of drug diffusion, and concentration equilibrium

Because of the factors discussed above, the speed with which capillary blood and tissue drug concentrations reach an equilibrium does not require only seconds as example 2.1 suggests. Instead it may take up to 10 minutes for intravascular-extravascular concentration equilibrium to be achieved for molecules whose molecular weight is less than 1000 g/mole [2,3,33,34]. Because fat-soluble molecules are less restricted in their movements, the speed with which this concentration equilibrium is achieved is very much more rapid for very fat-soluble drugs than for fat-insoluble drugs [3,6].

Blood flow and drug diffusion/transport

Drug transport to any tissue is directly proportional to tissue blood flow. The higher the blood flow to a tissue, the greater the rate of drug delivery to that tissue, and vice versa.

Diffusion-limited drug uptake

In tissues with a relatively high blood flow, e.g. brain, liver, heart etc, the rate with which a drug can enter those tissues is not limited by the rate at which that drug is delivered to the tissues. Instead it is limited by the rate at which that drug can diffuse out of the capillaries into those tissues. This situation is called **diffusion-limited uptake**.

Flow-limited drug uptake

The situation where flow of blood into a tissue limits drug uptake of drug into that tissue is called **flow-limited uptake**. There are two ways in which this can occur.

1.   Some drugs enter pericapillary tissues by means of active transport processes, e.g. transport of penicillins into renal tubules. The rate of drug transport by such processes may be so rapid that most of the drug entering the tissue concerned is removed in a single passage through the capillary bed of that tissue. In such a situation, transport of drug into the tissue by blood flow is the factor which limits drug entry into the tissue.

2.   Blood flow is relatively low in some tissues, e.g. adipose tissue. Some drugs can diffuse very rapidly through capillary endothelium to enter the pericapillary tissues. In such a situation, the rate at which a drug enters such tissues is limited by the rate at which blood flow delivers that drug to those tissues.

Relation of drug diffusion and blood flow to kinetics and dynamics

The kinetic and dynamic properties of a drug are directly related to the rate with which a drug is transported to tissues by blood, as well as the speed with which that drug can diffuse into and out of the pericapillary tissues.

Blood flow

Blood is the medium in which all drugs are transported to and from tissues.

- Rate of onset of drug effect is directly proportional to blood flow to effector tissues, e.g. as with gallamine [39].

- The rate at which drugs are transported and distributed throughout the body is directly proportional to the cardiac output. Distribution rate constants are directly related to tissue, organ or drug compartment blood flow [38].

- Most drugs enter pericapillary tissues by means of bulk flow and diffusion. When a drug enters pericapillary tissues, the drug within those tissues eventually reaches a concentration equilibrium with the same drug in the blood supplying those tissues. The speed with which a substance whose molecular weight is less than 1000 g/mole achieves a concentration equilibrium between capillary blood and the tissues in which the capillaries are situated has been found to be directly proportional to the tissue blood flow [33,34].

- Some tissues or organs may metabolize or excrete a drug extremely rapidly. In such situations, the rate at which flow of blood delivers such a drug to these organs or tissues is the factor that limits the rate of drug excretion and metabolism. Alfentanil [35] and lidocaine [36,37] are examples of such drugs. Both drugs undergo extensive hepatic metabolism and excretion. The rates at which both drugs are removed from the body are directly proportional to hepatic blood flow and cardiac output.

- Some drugs are metabolized or excreted very slowly. Even a low tissue or organ blood flow may be sufficient to deliver such a drug more rapidly than excretion or metabolism by an organ(s) can remove it from the body. Examples of such drugs are diazepam, tolbutamide and warfarin [37].

Diffusion

Diffusion is the principal process by which drugs are exchanged between extravascular tissues and capillary blood.

- The rate of onset and termination of drug effect in any given tissue is directly proportional to the speed with which drugs diffuse into or out of the perivascular tissues in which they are active.

- The volume throughout which a drug is distributed is directly related to the degree of fat-solubility of that drug. A fat soluble drug can readily diffuse out of capillaries and into pericapillary cells and interstitium. Fat-insoluble drugs are confined to the extracellular fluid volume because they cannot diffuse easily into cells.

• The volume throughout which a drug is distributed is directly related to the speed with which it diffuses into perivascular tissues relative to the rate of elimination of that drug from the body. For example if a drug is very fat soluble, but is eliminated very rapidly, the volume throughout which it is distributed will not be large because most of the drug will have been eliminated before diffusion causes significant extravascular drug distribution. A good example of such a drug is glyceryl trinitrate. On the other hand, if a drug is fat soluble but eliminated slowly, then the volume throughout which it is distributed is large because ample time is available for diffusion to widely distribute the drug before significant elimination has occurred. An example of such a drug is thiopental. The same considerations also apply to less fat-soluble drugs, although the volumes throughout which such drugs are distributed are generally smaller.

EFFECT OF HEART AND LUNGS ON DRUG KINETICS

Earlier parts of this chapter have discussed the relevance of cardiac output and tissue blood flow to drug distribution. However cardiac output and tissue blood flow are not the only factors of importance. The initial distribution, as well as the magnitude of the effects of many intravenously administered drugs are determined by cardiovascular anatomy and physiology. This section sets out to explain why cardiovascular anatomy and physiology are of importance in clinical pharmacokinetics.

Relevance of cardiovascular anatomy and physiology to clinical drug use

The relevance of cardiovascular anatomy and physiology to pharmacokinetics and dynamics is clearly demonstrated by the fact that current kinetic and dynamic models cannot explain a number of features of clinical anesthetic drug use.

• Drugs cannot diffuse out of veins, the cardiac chambers, or arteries. So any intravenously administered drug must first pass through the heart, lungs and arteries before entering the capillaries of any organ other than the lung. So regardless of how rapidly a drug is injected, it always takes a finite time before it arrives at any peripheral tissue after intravenous injection. All this is predicted by the circulation time concept, but is ignored by current pharmacokinetic models. These assume that drug distribution throughout any pharmacokinetic compartment is complete and instantaneous.

• The maximum volume of blood in which a single intravenous dose of a rapidly injected drug can possibly mix prior to emerging from the aortic valve is equal to the volume of venous blood entering heart during the injection period, plus the volume of blood in the pulmonary circulation and the heart chambers. This is about 1400 ml in the normal adult [40]. Therefore the blood concentration of a drug as it enters the aorta and arteries can initially be quite high. Such high initial drug concentrations are not predicted by current pharmacokinetic models.

- After intravenous drug injection, arterial drug concentrations are initially always higher than venous. This is a consequence of the fact that an intravenously administered drug must first pass through the heart, lungs and arterial system before entering any tissues and veins. Now when a drug passes through peripheral tissues, it can leave the blood by diffusion into these tissues through capillaries. Initially the arterial and capillary drug concentrations are much higher than the tissue drug concentrations, and so drug diffuses out of blood into tissues. This means that the venous concentration of a drug is initially always lower than the arterial concentration of that same drug. Indeed this is confirmed by studies which have shown that arterial drug concentrations are higher than venous concentrations for 2-4 minutes after intravenous injection [50,51]. Current pharmacokinetic models are frequently based only on data derived from measurement of venous blood drug concentrations. As a result they underestimate the arterial blood drug concentrations in the first few minutes after intravenous administration.

The above physiological facts have profound consequences for understanding the clinical effects of anesthetic drugs administered as a single rapid intravenous dose. Many drugs administered in this manner exert a clinically evident effect within 20-30 seconds after administration. Good examples of such drugs are the intravenous hypnotic drugs used for induction of anesthesia. When these drugs are administered rapidly intravenously, they cause cardiovascular and central nervous system depression within 20-30 seconds after administration. Kinetic-dynamic models based on data from intravenous drug concentration studies cannot predict such a rapid onset of action [see example 5.3 in chapter 5].

Physiologically based models of drug kinetics and dynamics are capable of describing all the phenomena observed with clinical drug use. However the facts of anatomy and physiology mean that physiological models are rather complex. Fortunately this complexity can be reduced somewhat by splitting the distribution of drugs within the body into various phases. To begin with, all drugs administered by the intravenous route must first pass through the heart and lungs before they reach any tissue where they are active. So it is useful to begin with a description of the effects of the heart and lungs on initial arterial drug concentrations. The way in which cardiopulmonary circulatory physiology determines initial arterial drug concentrations can be described with a model, which for lack of a better name can be called the "pre-recirculation" phase model.

The "pre-recirculation phase" defined

It takes some time for an intravenously or intra-atrially administered drug to arrive in the veins of the body. After such a drug has returned to the heart through the veins it recirculates, passing though the heart and into the arteries again. Table 2.1 gives an idea of how long it takes an intravenously administered drug to recirculate. The physiological fact of recirculation allows the definition of a new phase in drug kinetics, the **pre-recirculation phase**. The pre-recirculation phase begins when a drug is injected into a vein or the right atrium, and ends when recirculated drug containing blood, (mainly from the upper body), starts to enter the aorta. Table 2.1 shows that this phase will last up to 20-30 seconds in the average adult [see fig 2.5].

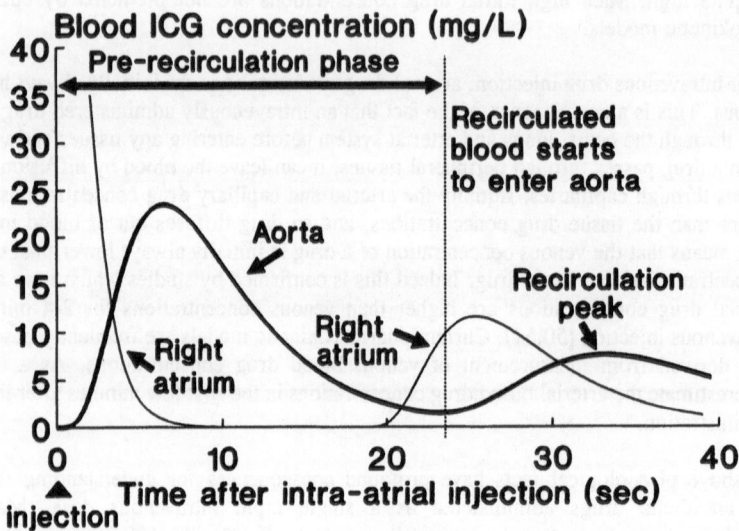

Figure 2.5: Simulated venous and aortic root blood concentration-time curves resulting from rapid injection of 20 mg indocyanine green (ICG) into the right atrium. The initial high aortic root ICG concentrations are the result of ICG passing through the heart and lungs for the first time, ("first pass"), and the second lower peak is due to passage of the ICG through the heart and lungs again after recirculation from the upper body.

Qualitative description of the effects of heart and lungs on drug kinetics

Cardiac chamber volumes and function, as well as pulmonary blood volume significantly affect the arterial drug concentrations achieved in the pre-recirculation phase.

Effect of right ventricle

Consider a drug which is infused at a constant rate into a peripheral vein or into the right atrium so that the drug concentration in the incoming blood is constant. Shortly after commencing drug administration, blood entering the right ventricle during diastole contains the drug. However the right ventricle is never totally emptied during systole. In fact about 50% of the volume of blood present in the right ventricle at the end of diastole is still present in the right ventricle at the end of systole. The fraction of the end-diastolic volume (EDV) that remains in the ventricle after ejection of the stroke volume (SV) is the **ejection fraction (EF)**. Ejection fraction is given by the formula **EF = SV/EDV**, and the EF of the right ventricle = 0.5 [12]. The concentration of the drug in blood entering the right ventricle is reduced by the blood remaining in the right ventricle. Turbulence of the blood contained in the right ventricle during diastole ensures nearly instantaneous and complete mixing of the incoming drug containing blood with the blood remaining in the right ventricle. During the next systole it is this drug solution which is pumped out. More drug containing blood enters the right ventricle during the next and subsequent diastolic phases. Now because some drug is already present, the drug concentration in the right ventricle is higher than in the previous cardiac cycle. The whole process repeats itself until the drug concentration in the right ventricle is the same as that in the atrial and venous blood [see example 1.1]. The situation is reversed when the blood entering the right ventricle no longer contains the drug [see example 1.2].

Effect of the pulmonary blood volume

Blood pumped out of the right ventricle must first pass through the pulmonary circulation before it enters the left atrium. There are two ways in which the pulmonary circulation may act on the drug in the blood passing through it.

- The drug may simply pass through the pulmonary vascular bed without mixing with blood present in the pulmonary vascular bed. Drug concentration in the blood entering the left atrium is then the same as in the right ventricle. This type of model is sometimes called the **parallel tube model.**

- A drug may behave as if it mixes with the pulmonary blood volume. This type of model is called the **well-stirred model.**

Experiment has shown that drugs passing through the pulmonary circulation behave as if they mix with the pulmonary blood volume [8,9,10,11]. So the "well-stirred" model is applicable in this situation.

Molecular weights of all the commonly used anesthetic drugs are less than 1000 g/mole. The pulmonary circulation is quite permeable to molecules such as albumin [13,14] whose molecular weight is 66241 g/mole. So it is not surprising that pulmonary capillaries readily permit the extravasation of anesthetic drugs. Because of this, the percentage of a given drug dose which diffuses into pulmonary interstitium during even a single passage through human lungs may be a significant fraction of the dose administered [see table 2.2]. Diffusion of drug into pulmonary interstitium has two effects.

- Less drug enters the left ventricle after passage through the lungs. This means that the concentration of that drug in the left ventricle, and eventually the aorta, is reduced.

- During a single passage through the lung, drug leaves the pulmonary capillaries if the intracapillary drug concentrations are higher than the pulmonary interstitial fluid drug concentrations. When the pulmonary capillary drug concentration falls below that in the pulmonary interstitial fluid, then drug diffuses back into the pulmonary capillaries. This has the effect of prolonging the time it takes all of a single dose of a drug to pass through the pulmonary vascular system.

Table 2.2.
Percentage of a single intravenous dose of various drugs diffusing into
lung tissue during a single passage though human lungs.

Drug	M.W. (g/mole)	% Drug dose diffusing into lung tissue in first pass
Indocyanine-green[8,9,11]	774	0%
Diazepam[7]	284.76	33.8%
Thiopental[7]	264.33	15.8%
Lidocaine[7]	234	60.5%
Meperidine[8]	247.34	64.5%
Morphine[8]	285.3	33.5%
Fentanyl[8,10]	336.46	75.2%
Alfentanil[9]	471	53.7%

Left ventricle

The left ventricle is filled with blood that has initially passed through the right ventricle and the pulmonary vascular system. Otherwise the effect of the left ventricle on initial arterial blood concentrations of any drug is almost precisely the same as for the right ventricle. The differences are that the left ventricle normally has an ejection fraction of about 0.67 and empties into the arterial system [see also examples 1.1 and 1.2].

Quantitative heart and lungs kinetic model

The whole system may now be described quantitatively. This may be done by using the above qualitative description of the multicompartment pharmacokinetic model of the heart and lungs depicted in figure 2.6a. Chapter 1 describes the method of deriving the systems of equations necessary to derive the rates of change of drug concentration in each compartment. These methods have been used to derive the equations describing the model depicted in figure 2.6b [17].

Consider the right ventricle, left ventricle, and pulmonary blood volume. Blood flows into the right ventricle at the same rate as it flows out. The same consideration applies to the pulmonary blood volume and the left ventricle. However the volumes of each of these three compartments is different. This means that their rate constants are also different. The rate constant in such a mechanical model is equal to the flow divided by the compartment volume [see chapter 1 for explanation]. So the input and output rate constants for each compartment are given by equations 2.4, 2.5 and 2.6.

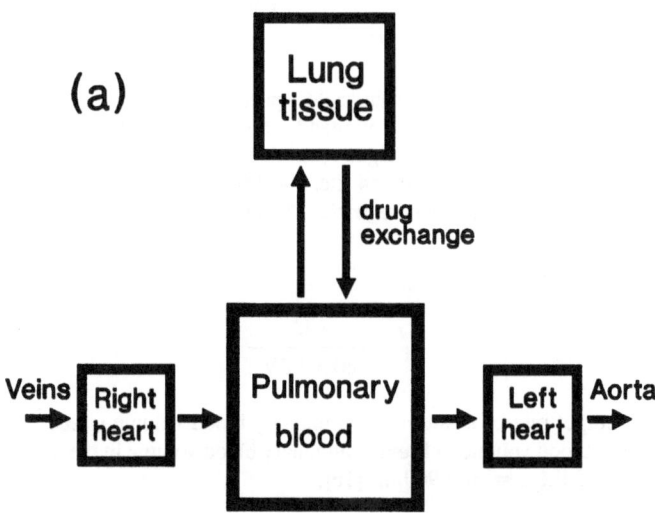

Figure 2.6: Figure 2.6a shows a physiological pharmacokinetic model of the heart and lungs. The right ventricle feeds the pulmonary vascular system, which in turn feeds the left ventricle, and also exchanges drug with lung tissue. Rate constants binding the left and right hearts with the pulmonary circulation have only one thing in common. The blood flow through all three is the same, and is equal to the cardiac output. Accordingly the right and left hearts are each considered as 1-compartment systems, while the lungs may be considered as a 2-compartment system [figure 2.6b].

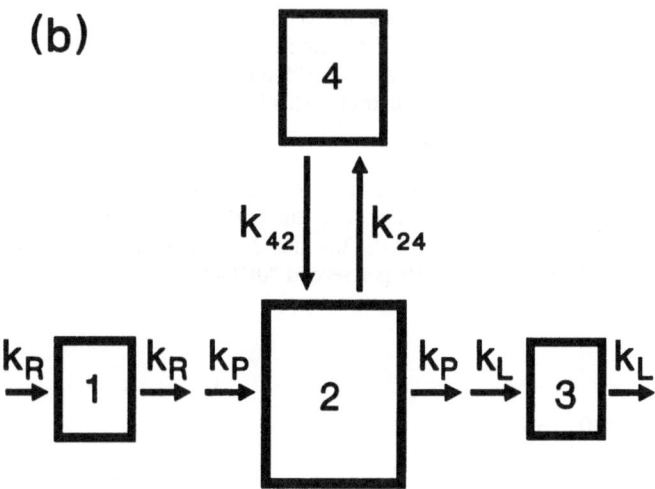

$$k_R = \frac{CO}{60 \times RVEDV} = \frac{HR \times RVEF}{60} \tag{2.4}$$

k_R is the input and output rate constant of the right ventricle in **sec^{-1}**.
CO is the cardiac output in **L/min**. This is divided by 60 to give cardiac output in **L/sec**.
RVEDV is the end diastolic volume of the right ventricle in **liters**. The end diastolic volume of the healthy right ventricle in adults is about 0.164 liters = 164 ml [12].
RVEF is the ejection fraction of the right ventricle. The usual value of the RVEF in healthy adults is 0.51 [12].
HR is the heart rate in **beats/minute**.

$$k_P = \frac{CO}{60 \times PBV} \tag{2.5}$$

k_P is the input and output rate constant of the pulmonary blood volume in **sec^{-1}**.
PBV is the pulmonary blood volume in **liters**. Pulmonary blood volume in the average healthy adult varies between 0.38-0.9 liters = 380-900 ml [16].

The fraction of a drug dose diffusing into pulmonary interstitium during a single passage of a drug through the pulmonary circulation differs from one drug to another, even for drugs having similar molecular weights [see table 2.2]. So the rate constants k_{24} and k_{42} must be experimentally determined. They describe drug exchange rates between the pulmonary blood volume and lung tissue.

$$k_L = \frac{CO}{60 \times LVEDV} = \frac{HR \times LVEF}{60} \tag{2.6}$$

k_L is the input and output rate constant of the left ventricle in **sec^{-1}**.
LVEDV is the end diastolic volume of the left ventricle in **liters**. The end diastolic volume of the left ventricle in healthy adults is normally about 0.125 liters = 125 ml [15].
LVEF is the ejection fraction of the left ventricle. This is usually 0.67 in a healthy adult [15].

Drug concentrations in compartments 1 to 4 are represented by C_1, C_2, C_3 and C_4 respectively. C_{in} is the concentration of the drug entering the right ventricle. The unit of drug concentration is mg/L. Equations 2.7, 2.8, 2.9 and 2.10 give the rates of change of drug concentration in each of the compartments per second "dC/dt".

Right ventricle

$$\frac{dC_1}{dt} = k_R(C_{in} - C_1) \tag{2.7}$$

Pulmonary blood volume

$$\frac{dC_2}{dt} = k_P(C_1 - C_2) + k_{42}.C_4 - k_{24}.C_2 \tag{2.8}$$

Pulmonary tissue

$$\frac{dC_4}{dt} = k_{24}.C_2 - k_{42}.C_4 \tag{2.9}$$

Left ventricular and Arterial drug concentrations

$$\frac{dC_3}{dt} = k_L(C_2 - C_3) \tag{2.10}$$

These equations may be solved using Euler's method [see chapter 1]. An example of the application of these equations is given in figure 2.7 for actual experimental data using indocyanine green. Indocyanine green is a substance, which for all practical purposes, does not diffuse out of lung capillaries to enter into lung tissue. This means that equation 2.9 need not be used.

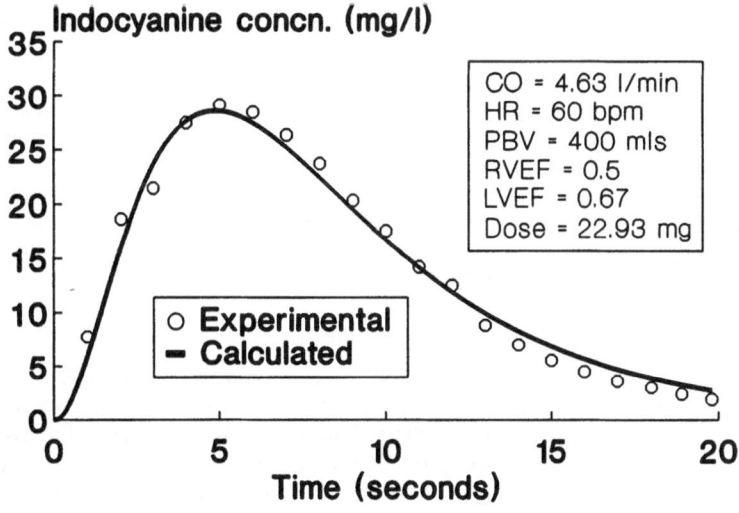

Figure 2.7: Pre-recirculation phase theoretical and experimental aortic root blood concentration-time curves for a dose of indocyanine green which was injected in less than 0.5 second into the right atrium at time = 0 seconds, (unpublished data of Dr F.Boer [18]).

General principles determining peak pre-recirculation phase drug concentration

It is useful to formulate some general rules which determine the magnitude and speed of occurrence of the pre-recirculation phase drug concentration peak.

- Time to pre-recirculation phase peak drug concentration is inversely proportional to cardiac output.

- Peak pre-recirculation phase drug concentration is directly proportional to the left and right ventricular ejection fractions.

- Peak pre-recirculation phase drug concentration is inversely proportional to the pulmonary blood volume.

Clinical implications of pre-recirculation phase peak drug concentration.

Pre-recirculation phase kinetics are of most importance for drugs which can rapidly diffuse into organs, e.g. the fat soluble intravenous hypnotic agents. This is simply because only such drugs can diffuse into tissues and organs in sufficient quantity to cause clinical effects in the short time that the pre-recirculation phase lasts. Pre-recirculation kinetics are of less importance for drugs which diffuse very slowly into pericapillary tissues, as only small and clinically insignificant amounts can enter any effector organ or tissue during the pre-recirculation phase, eg. some opiates and non-depolarizing muscle relaxants.

There are two important aspects to the peak pre-recirculation phase drug concentration, the speed with which the concentration peak occurs, and the concentration achieved.

- The sooner the pre-recirculation phase peak drug concentration occurs, the sooner the drug will act. Speed of arrival of a drug at any tissue or organ is determined by circulation time, and circulation time is inversely related to cardiac output.

- The greater the pre-recirculation phase peak drug concentration, the greater the magnitude of the drug effect exerted by drugs which rapidly diffuse into tissues, eg. drugs used as intravenous induction agents in anesthesia.

Pre-recirculation phase in various clinical situations

The heart-lung model developed in the last few pages can be used to explain a number of drug effects in various common clinical situations. These are simulated in this section. Several assumptions have been made when making these simulations. The percentage of a given dose of a drug that diffuses into lung tissue during the first passage through the pulmonary circulation is assumed to be constant for a given drug regardless of the clinical circumstances. Effects of changes of each of the individual parameters used in this model are also not shown as isolated changes of each of these parameters never occurs. A change of any one of the parameters in this model is always associated with a change of another of the variables.

Figure 2.8: Simulated pre-recirculation phase concentration-time curves resulting from rapid intravenous administration of a 10 mg dose of a drug to normal persons, and to persons who are anxious or receiving inotropic drugs.

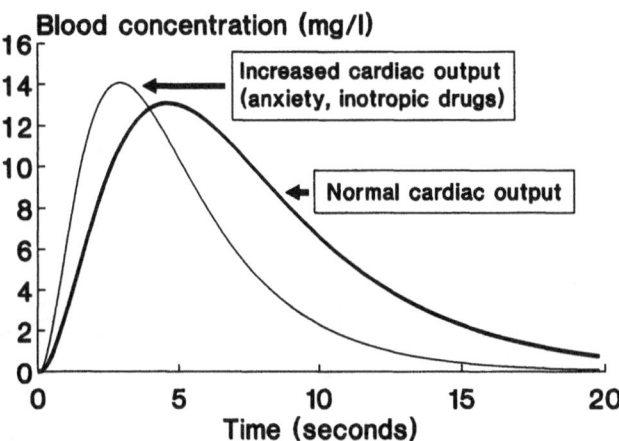

Tachycardia due to a cardiac pacemaker

Tachycardia may be induced by a cardiac pacemaker. Such a tachycardia induces no changes in cardiac function except to increase the heart rate. Cardiac output is unchanged from that at normal rates until the heart rate exceeds 150 beats/min, after which it decreases [45]. So at heart rates below 150 beats per minute, cardiac output, right and left ventricular ejection fractions and pulmonary blood volume are unchanged from their rest values, despite rate related reductions of end-systolic and end-diastolic ventricular volumes [46]. This means that neither the time of onset, not the pre-recirculation phase peak drug concentration are affected by pacing induced tachycardia below 150 beats/minute, (k_R , k_P and k_L remain normal).

Anxiety and inotropic drugs

Cardiac pacemakers are a very infrequent cause of tachycardiac in clinical practice. Usually tachycardia is due to either inotropic drugs or increased sympathetic nervous activity due to anxiety. Both anxiety [49] and inotropic drugs [47,48] increase right and left ventricular ejection fractions, heart rate and cardiac output, while leaving pulmonary blood volume relatively unchanged.

Increased cardiac output reduces circulation times between all points of the body, and so the time to occurrence of the pre-recirculation phase peak drug concentration is shortened. Because the cardiac output relative to the pulmonary blood volume, as well as the ventricular ejection fractions are increased, the magnitude of the peak pre-recirculation phase drug concentration is increased too, (i.e. k_R , k_P and k_L are increased). This situation has been simulated in figure 2.8.

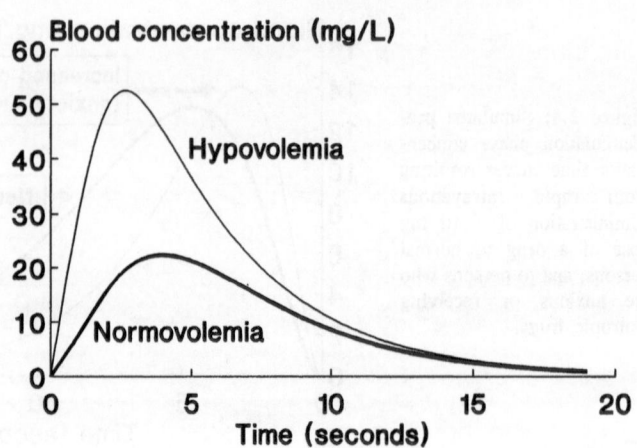

Figure 2.9: Simulated pre-recirculation phase concentration-time curves resulting from rapid intravenous administration of a 10 mg dose of a drug to normovolemic and severely hypovolemic persons.

Hypovolemia and pre-recirculation phase kinetics

Significant hypovolemia, defined as loss of more than 10-15% of the blood volume, is associated with profound hemodynamic effects. End-diastolic volumes of both ventricles, cardiac output, blood pressure and pulmonary blood volume [44] are reduced below normal levels. The ejection fractions of both ventricles and the heart rate are increased above normal levels. Of all these changes, the most significant is the reduction of pulmonary blood volume to such a degree that pre-recirculation phase drug concentrations are increased above normal, (increased k_P, and possibly k_L and k_R) [52]. The effects of these changes on the pre-recirculation phase blood drug concentrations are compared in figure 2.9 for the same dose of the same drug administered to normovolemic and hypovolemic persons.

Physical exertion and pre-recirculation phase drug kinetics

Physical exertion has a profound effect on cardiac and hemodynamic function. The main changes are that heart rate, cardiac output, and the ejection fractions of both ventricles increase [43], while pulmonary blood volume increases only minimally, (about 16%), above the resting level [42]. Increased cardiac output means that the pre-recirculation phase peak drug concentration occurs sooner than in resting persons. In addition the magnitude of the pre-recirculation phase peak drug concentration is increased above resting levels because of the increased ventricular ejection fractions, together with a cardiac output elevation relative to the pulmonary blood volume, (increased k_R, k_P and k_L). These changes have been simulated in figure 2.10.

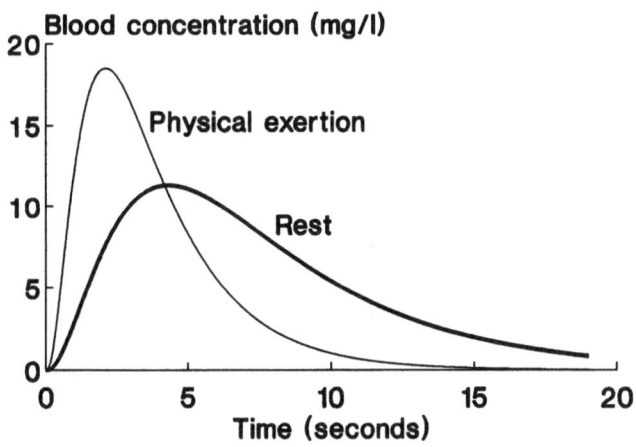

Figure 2.10: Simulated pre-recirculation phase concentration-time curves resulting from rapid intravenous administration of a 10 mg dose of a drug to resting adults, and to adults undertaking physical exertion.

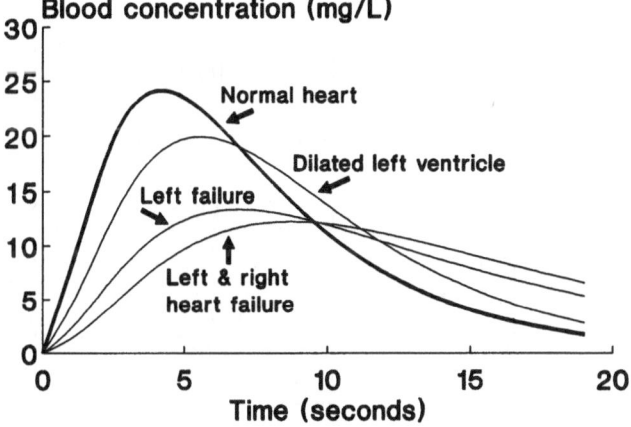

Figure 2.11: Simulated pre-recirculation phase concentration-time curves resulting from rapid intravenous administration of a 10 mg dose of a drug to normal adults, and to adults with various types of cardiac dysfunction.

Pre-recirculation phase drug kinetics and disorders of ventricular function

Figure 2.11 compares the pre-recirculation phase drug concentrations for the situation where an identical drug dose has been administered to persons with various types of cardiac dysfunction. The situations simulated are those of a normal cardiovascular system, left ventricular dilation, left ventricular failure, and combined right and left ventricular failure.

- Isolated left ventricular dilation can occur without being associated with cardiac failure or increased pulmonary blood volume. The only significant change is a reduction of the left ventricular ejection fraction and increased left ventricular end diastolic volume. Reduction of the left ventricular ejection fraction reduces the magnitude of the peak pre-recirculation phase drug concentration, (reduced k_L).

- Left ventricular failure is characterized by reduced cardiac output and left ventricular ejection fraction, together with increased left ventricular end diastolic volume and pulmonary blood volume. A reduced cardiac output delays the occurrence of the peak pre-recirculation phase drug concentration, while increased pulmonary blood volume, reduced cardiac output and left ventricular ejection fraction all combine to reduce the magnitude of the pre-recirculation phase peak drug concentration, (decreased k_P and k_L).

- Failure of both right and left ventricles has essentially the same effect as failure of the left ventricle alone, only the right ventricular ejection fraction is also reduced. This means that the changes of pre-recirculation phase kinetics are even more pronounced than for left ventricular failure alone, (reduced k_R, k_P and k_L).

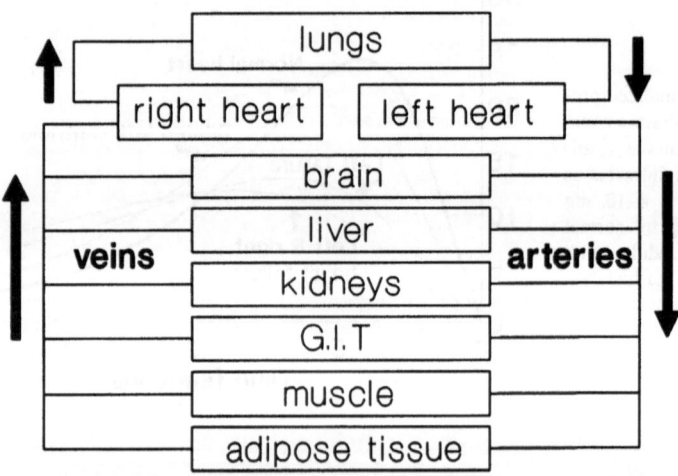

Figure 2.12: The arterial system transports the blood and drugs within it to all the organs and tissues of the body. Veins drain the blood and transport it back to the heart. Organs and tissues may be considered to be fed and drained in parallel. Blood drug concentration in the artery of each organ is the same. The only exception to this rule is the pulmonary artery. Blood drug concentrations in the veins draining each organ or tissue may be quite different due to differing drug uptake by each organ or tissue.

PHYSIOLOGICAL PHARMACOKINETIC MODELS

Once an intravenously administered drug enters the arterial system it is distributed by the arteries to all the organs and tissues of the body, [see figure 2.12]. Each of the organs and tissues of the body has a different size and blood flow per unit weight [see table 2.3].

Figure 2.12 and table 2.3 show that each organ or tissue can be considered as a functional pharmacokinetic drug compartment. Such compartments have already been discussed in chapter 1, and the heart and lungs have already been treated in this way in this chapter. A physiological pharmacokinetic model consists of a whole series of equations, where each compartment is described by one or more equations. Such pharmacokinetic models have been constructed [19]. These models are often quite complex because of the number of equations required. Fortunately, with the current ready availability of cheap and powerful microcomputers, complex series of equations present no real objection to the use of such kinetic models. However any practical use of these models is at present associated with several problems.

Table 2.3.

Organ	Organ weight (% body weight)	Organ flow (% cardiac output)	Organ flow (ml/100 gm /minute)	IFV (% organ weight)
Lungs	1.6[20]	>95	540[20]	50[23,41]
Liver	2[20]	28	100[26,27]	16[41]
Kidneys	0.5[20]	23	340[20,28]	35[41]
Skeletal muscle	43[20]	16	10-12[29]	12[24,41]
Brain	2.3[20]	14	50[30]	22[25,41]
Skin	7[20]	9	11[20]	50[24,41]
Heart	0.4[20]	5	69[31]	8-20[24]
Adipose tissue	16-36[21,22]	<5	2-7[32]	18[41]

IFV = Interstitial Fluid Volume.

Problems with the use of physiological models

The problems currently facing the physiological pharmacokinetic models essentially stem from two sources, lack of data, and lack of technical capability to measure essential parameters.

- A solid organ or tissue is not the same as the chambers of the heart. Drug diffuses out of capillaries into the interstitium and cells of a solid organ or tissue. The diffusion rate of a drug through any capillary or tissue is determined by factors such as capillary pore size, drug molecular weight, degree of ionization, and fat-solubility. This means that each drug and tissue must be treated individually. Diffusion constants for each organ and tissue are simply unknown for most anesthetic drugs.

- The solubility of most anesthetic drugs within the major organs of the body is unknown for most drugs. A notable exception to this rule is the extensive body of data on the tissue and organ solubilities of inhalational anesthetic drugs.

- The volume in which a drug mixes within each tissue or organ is technically difficult to define and measure. In addition to this, organ sizes vary from one individual to another.

- The average resting blood flow through most organs and tissues is known. However organ blood flow varies quite considerably even under normal physiological conditions. In addition to this, blood flow also changes in response to anesthetic drugs, anesthetic techniques, surgery, pain and psychological factors. These changes in tissue and organ flow are technically difficult to measure.

It is evident from these few points that physiological pharmacokinetic models, while attractive because of their physiological basis, are relatively useless in practice. Essential data are either lacking or deficient. In addition to these problems, variation in normal anatomy, physiology and function means that the use of averaged data yields relatively inaccurate results in any one individual. Consequently empirical models are usually used to describe drug kinetics.

Empirical pharmacokinetic models have the advantage of being mathematically less complex than genuinely physiologically based models. They are also based on data which are much easier to collect, as well as being just as accurate as physiological models in terms of the predictions able to be made with them [19].

EMPIRICAL MULTICOMPARTMENT PHARMACOKINETIC MODELS

The process of developing an empirical pharmacokinetic model is as follows. A drug is administered. Blood is sampled at intervals after administration, and the drug concentration is measured in these samples. A blood drug concentration-time curve is the result. The drug concentration-time curve can be described with a mathematical equation. This equation is purely a description of the experimental findings. A model can then be devised which will give rise to such an equation. Such a model need not have any anatomical or physiological basis.

Most current pharmacokinetic models are derived in just this way, and are accordingly empirical pharmacokinetic models. Because of the anatomy and physiology of the body they are usually multicompartment models.

Empirically determined drug concentration-time curves

The blood drug concentration-time curves resulting from a single intravenous administration of a drug are sometimes able to be described with a monoexponential decay equation. More usually these curves are best able to be described with bi-exponential or tri-exponential decay equations.

This is surprising. The expected result would be that the blood concentration-time curve would be the product of drug entry and exit from each compartment, i.e. each different organ or tissue of the body. Each compartment would have its own rate of entry and exit for a given drug. This can be described for each compartment with a mono-exponential equation. The equation describing the blood concentration-time curve resulting from a single rapid intravenous injection of a drug, would therefore be expected to have as many exponential terms as there are compartments or major organ or tissue groups, i.e. at least 5 exponential terms [see fig. 2.12]. However this is not so. Only one, two or three exponential terms are required in the equations. So the body may be considered from a pharmacokinetic viewpoint to be composed of one, two or three drug containing compartments respectively.

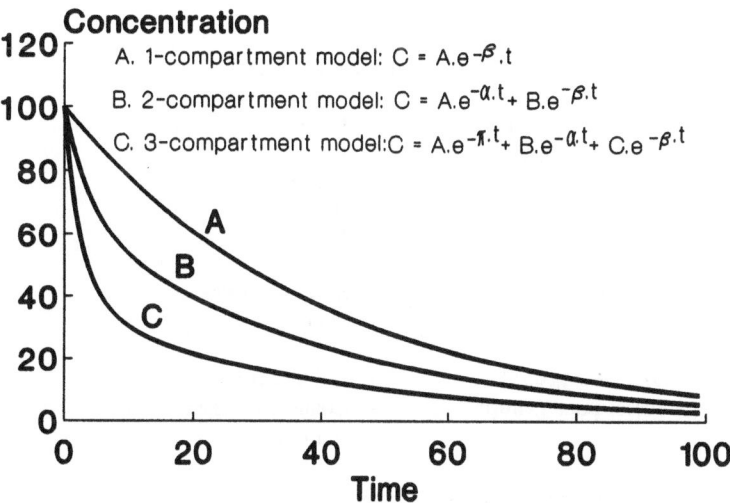

Figure 2.13: Mono-, bi- and tri-exponential blood drug concentration time curves which may result from the intravenous administration of a single dose of a drug.

Table 2.4.

Organs may be classified as to their blood flow relative to their total weight. Organs with a blood flow which is high in relation to their total weight are called "high flow" or "vessel rich", and the reverse is true for those with a blood flow which is low in relation to their weight.

TWO COMPARTMENTS

"High flow group"	- Lungs
"Vessel rich group"	- Liver
	- Kidneys
	- Brain
	- Heart
"Low flow group"	- Skeletal muscle
"Vessel poor group"	- Adipose tissue
	- Skin
	- Connective tissue
	and bone

THREE COMPARTMENTS

"High flow group"	- Lungs
"Vessel rich group"	- Liver
	- Kidneys
	- Brain
	- Heart
"Medium flow group"	- Skeletal muscle
	- Skin
"Low flow group"	- Adipose tissue
"Vessel-poor group"	- Connective tissue
	and bone

Drugs whose decay curve may be described by a mono-exponential decay equation are not common. The implication of a mono-exponential decay curve is that the body may be considered as a single pharmacokinetic compartment for some drugs, and means that the rate at which a drug can enter and leave all organs and tissues of the body is the same.

The decay curves of many drugs may be described by a bi-exponential equation, meaning that the drug behaves as if it is distributed throughout two functional pharmacokinetic compartments. One compartment into which the drug can enter and leave rapidly, and a second compartment in which the rate of drug entry and departure is much slower. Tables 2.3 and 2.4 show that this may be accounted for by the fact that some tissues have a relatively high blood flow in relation to the cardiac output. These are the "vessel-rich group" of tissues, and these comprise the rapid compartment. Other tissues may be considered as "low flow", or "vessel-poor" tissues or organs. This latter group of tissues comprise the slower compartment.

Curves which are described by a tri-exponential equation may be accounted for by dividing the body into tissues where the blood flow is high, medium or low [see tables 2.3 and 2.4].

Drug transport into, and out of compartments

A drug is transported from one part of the body to another by blood. Drugs diffuse from the blood into organs and tissues, and in the reverse direction too. This corresponds to transport of drug into and out of pharmacokinetic compartments.

Cardiac output and empirical pharmacokinetic models

Blood flow to each organ and groups of organs or tissues is directly related to cardiac output, see table 2.3]. As each of the compartments in these empirical models is related to groups of tissues with differing relative blood flows, it is only to be expected that the rates at which a drug enters into, and is exchanged between these empirically determined compartments are directly related to the cardiac output. This has indeed been found to been the case for alfentanil, where the intercompartmental rate constants have been found to be directly related to cardiac output [38].

Use of empirical pharmacokinetic models

The empirical multicompartment models are the most commonly used pharmacokinetic models at present. They form the subject matter of the next chapter.

CONCLUDING REMARKS

The purpose of this chapter has been to give a view of the physiological basis of current multi-compartment pharmacokinetic models, and pharmacodynamics. One of the main reasons for this discussion is the author's belief that an understanding of the physiological basis of these models provides a more intuitive understanding of the rather more abstract concepts to be introduced in the following two chapters.

REFERENCES

1.   Altman PL, et al.,(eds.),"Handbook of Circulation", pub. W.B. Saunders, U.S.A., 1959, Library of Congress No. 59-15183, pages 115-125.
2.   Pappenheimer JR, et al: Filtration, diffusion and molecular sieving through peripheral capillary membranes. *American Journal of Physiology*, 1951: 167: 13-46.
3.   Pappenheimer JR: Passage of molecules through capillary walls. *Physiological Reviews*, 1953: 33: 387-423.
4.   Woerlee GM,"Common Perioperative Problems and the Anaesthetist", published Kluwer Academic Publishers, the Netherlands, 1988, ISBN 0-89838-402-8, pages 508-510.
5.   Apelblat A, et al: A mathematical analysis of capillary-tissue fluid exchange. *Biorheology*, 1974: 11: 1-49.
6.   Renkin EM: Capillary permeability to lipid-soluble molecules. *American Journal of Physiology*, 1952: 168: 538-545.
7.   Kotrly KJ, et al: First pass uptake of lidocaine, diazepam, and thiopental in the human lung. *Anesthesia and Analgesia*, 1988: 67: S119.
8.   Roerig DK, et al: First pass uptake of fentanyl, meperidine, and morphine in the human lung. *Anesthesiology*, 1987: 67: 466-472.
9.   Taeger K, et al: Pulmonary kinetics of fentanyl and alfentanil in surgical patients. *British Journal of Anaesthesia*, 1988: 61: 425-434.
10. Taeger K, et al: Uptake of fentanyl by human lung. *Anesthesiology*, 1984: 61: A246.
11. Weigand BD, et al: The use of indocyanine green for the evaluation of hepatic function and blood flow in man. *American Journal of Digestive Diseases*, 1960: 5: 427-436
12. Gentzler RD, et al: Angiographic estimation of right ventricular volume in man. *Circulation*, 1974: 50: 324-330.
13. McNamee JE, Staub NC: Pore models of sheep lung microvascular barrier using new data on protein tracers. *Microvascular Research*, 1979: 18: 229-224.
14. Brigham KL, Owen PJ: Mechanism of the serotonin effect on lung transvascular fluid and protein movement in awake sheep. *Circulation Research*, 1975: 36: 761-770.
15. Kennedy JW, et al: Quantitative angiography. I. The normal left ventricle in man. *Circulation*, 1966: 34: 272-278.
16. Slutsky R, et al: Pulmonary blood volume. Correlation of equilibrium radionucleotide and dye-dilution estimates. *Investigative Radiology*, 1982: 17: 233-240.
17. This model was developed by Dr F. Boer together with the author. Dr F. Boer is an anesthesiologist in the Department of Anesthesiology of the University Hospital of Leiden, Leiden, the Netherlands, (Head of Department, Prof. Dr. J. Spierdijk).
18. Unpublished data of Dr F. Boer. The post-injection indocyanine green dye curves were obtained as part of a preliminary pilot study of this model.
19. Wagner JG: "Fundamentals of Clinical Pharmacokinetics", pub. Drug Intelligence Publications Inc., U.S.A, ISBN 0-914678-20-4, pages 124-125.
20. Diem,K., Lentner,C.,"Wissenschaftliche Tabellen", 7th edn., pub. CIBA-GEIGY A.G., Basel, 1968.
21. Bruce A, et al: Body composition. Prediction of normal body potassium, body water and body fat in adults on the basis of body height, body weight and age. *Scandinavian Journal of Clinical & Laboratory Investigation*, 1980: 40: 461-473.
22. Moore FD, et al, "The Body Cell Mass and its Supporting Environment. Body Composition in Health and Disease.", published W.B.Saunders Co., U.S.A., 1963, pages 167-168.
23. Staub NC: Pulmonary edema. *Physiological Reviews*, 1974: 54: 678-811.

24. Aukland K, Nicolaysen G: Interstitial fluid volume: Local regulatory mechanisms. *Physiological Reviews*, 1981: 61: 556-643.
25. Holliday MA, et al: Factors that limit brain volume changes in response to acute and sustained hyper- and hyponatremia. *Journal of Clinical Investigation*, 1968: 47: 1916-1928.
26. Wiegand BD, et al: The use of indocyanine green for the evaluation of hepatic function and blood flow in man. *American Journal of Digestive Diseases*, 1960: 5: 427-436.
27. Caesar J, et al: The use of indocyanine green in the measurement of hepatic blood flow and as a test of hepatic function. *Clinical Science*, 1961: 21: 43-57.
28. Goldring W, et al: Relations of effective renal blood flow and glomerular function to tubular excretory mass in normal man. *Journal of Clinical Investigation*, 1940: 19: 739-750.
29. Evans EF, et al: Blood flow in muscle groups and drug absorption. *Clinical Pharmacology & Therapeutics*, 1975: 17: 44-47.
30. Lassen NA: Cerebral blood flow and oxygen consumption in man. *Physiological Reviews*, 1959: 39: 183-238.
31. Johnson LL, et al: Reduced left ventricular myocardial blood flow per unit mass in aortic stenosis. *Circulation*, 1978: 57: 582-590.
32. Lesser GT, Deutsch S: Measurement of adipose tissue flow and perfusion in man by uptake of $^{85}K^1$. *Journal of Applied Physiology*, 1967: 23: 621-630.
33. Landis EM, Pappenheimer JR: Exchange of substances through the capillary walls. in "Handbook of Physiology", section 2, "Circulation", volume II, eds. Hamilton WF and Dow P, pub. American Physiological Society, Washington D.C., 1963.
34. Renkin EM: Effects of blood flow on diffusion kinetics in isolated perfused hindlegs of cats. *American Journal of Physiology*, 1955: 183: 125-136.
35. Chauvin M, et al: The influence of hepatic plasma flow on alfentanil plasma concentration plateaus achieved with an infusion model in humans: Measurement of alfentanil hepatic extraction coefficient. *Anesthesia and Analgesia*, 1986: 65: 999-1003.
36. Stenson RE, et al: Interrelationships of hepatic blood flow, cardiac output, and blood levels of lidocaine in man. *Circulation*, 1971: 43: 205-211.
37. Nies AS, et al: Altered hepatic blood flow and drug disposition. *Clinical Pharmacokinetics*, 1976: 1: 135-155.
38. Krejcie TC, et al: Alfentanil pharmacokinetics: Intravascular space and cardiac output. *Anesthesiology*, 1988: 69: A466.
39. Goat VA, et al: The effect of blood flow upon the activity of gallamine triethiodide. *British Journal of Anaesthesia*, 1976: 48: 69-73.
40. London GM, et al: Cardiopulmonary blood volume and plasma renin activity in normal and hypertensive humans. *American Journal of Physiology*, 1985: 249: H807-H813.
41. Pierson RN, et al: Extracellular water measurements:organ tracer kinetics of bromide and sucrose in rats and man. *American Journal of Physiology*, 1978: 235: F254-F264.
42. Slutsky RA, et al: Pulmonary blood volume: Analysis during exercise in patients with left ventricular dysfunction. *European Journal of Nuclear Medicine*, 1983: 8: 523-527.
43. Maddahi J, et al: What is the normal range for left and right ventricular ejection fraction at different levels of exercise? Findings of scintgraphic ventriculography during graded ergometry in 34 normals. *Journal of Nuclear Medicine*, 1980: 21: P5.
44. Mangano DT, et al: The effect of increasing preload on ventricular output and ejection in man. Limitations of the Frank-Starling mechanism. *Circulation*, 1980: 62: 535-541.
45. Ross J, et al: Effects of changing heart rate in man by electrical stimulation of the right atrium. *Circulation*, 1965: 32: 549-558.

46.   Firth BG, et al: Effect of increasing heart rate in patients with aortic regurgitation. Effect of incremental atrial pacing on scintigraphic, hemodynamic and thermodilution measurements. *American Journal of Cardiology*, 1982: 49: 1860-1867.

47.   Slutsky R, et al: Left ventricular size and function after subcutaneous administration of terbutaline. Assessment by cardiac pool imaging. *Chest*, 1981: 79: 501-505.

48.   Hurwitz RA, et al: Dobutamine infusion to assess ventricular function in pediatric patients. *Journal of Nuclear Medicine*, 1987: 28: 621.

49.   Kiess MC, et al: Changes in ventricular function during emotional stress and cold exposure. *Journal of Nuclear Medicine*, 1984: 25: P4.

50.   Barratt RL, et al: Kinetics of thiopentone in relation to the site of sampling. *British Journal of Anaesthesia*, 1984: 56: 1385-1391.

51.   Major E, et al: Influence of sample site on blood concentrations of ICI 35 868. *British Journal of Anaesthesia*, 1983: 55: 371-375.

52.   Conn HL, Goldberg J: Accuracy of a radiopotassium dilution (Stewart principle) method for the measurement of cardiac output. *Journal of Applied Physiology*, 1955: 7: 542-548.

Chapter 3

Multicompartment Kinetic Models

Chapter 2 discussed the basic physiological principles underlying multicompartment pharmacokinetic models while chapter 1 reviewed the basic methods of their mathematical treatment. This chapter will discuss the principles of these models further. Multicompartment models are currently preferred for two important reasons. The data required are readily derived from measurements of blood drug concentrations. Secondly, multicompartment models are not as mathematically complex, and yet yield predictions which are as accurate as those made by physiological models.

This chapter is divided into two parts. The first part discusses properties common to all multicompartment models, while the second part discusses one-, two- and three-compartment models. Most emphasis in this book is placed on the 2-compartment model. This is because the 2-compartment model is physiologically realistic, as well as being usable in the clinical situation.

METHODS OF EXPRESSING DRUG CONCENTRATION

There are a number of methods of expressing drug concentration in various body tissues.

Blood drug concentration

Blood drug concentration is the concentration of a drug in whole blood measured after hemolysis of the erythrocytes. This measurement takes no account of whether the drug is present inside the erythrocytes or not. It also takes no account of whether there is any difference between the erythrocyte and plasma concentrations. It is simply a measure of the average drug concentration in both plasma and erythrocytes in a sample of whole blood.

Plasma drug concentration

Plasma drug concentration is the concentration of a drug in plasma only, regardless of whether that drug is also present inside erythrocytes.

Serum drug concentration

Serum is plasma from which coagulation proteins have been removed by allowing the blood to coagulate. Drug concentration in serum may differ from that measured in plasma because of the absence of coagulation proteins.

Erythrocyte drug concentration

A drug which is present in plasma may also diffuse inside the erythrocytes. The amount of drug present inside erythrocytes may actually be a significant fraction of the total amount of drug present in blood. Drug present inside leukocytes my be ignored, as the volume of leukocytes inside a given blood volume is negligible. Erythrocyte drug concentration is usually expressed as the ratio of the erythrocyte drug concentration divided by the plasma concentration of the same drug. This is called the **erythrocyte/plasma partition coefficient**. Erythrocyte/plasma partition coefficients of various anesthetic drugs are listed in appendix-B.

Tissue drug concentration

Drugs are not only present in blood, but are present inside extravascular tissues too. The concentrations of drugs inside extravascular tissues are usually given as the ratio of the exsanguinated whole tissue drug concentration divided by the simultaneously measured plasma concentration. This is the **tissue/plasma partition coefficient**. Appendix-B lists the partition coefficients of various anesthetic drugs in muscle, brain, and adipose tissue.

BASIC PROPERTIES OF PHARMACOKINETIC COMPARTMENTS

The basic properties of a pharmacokinetic compartment have already been defined in chapter 1. These are repeated below.

A pharmacokinetic compartment is a volume into, and out of which drug flows. Once in the compartment a drug is considered to be instantly and homogeneously distributed throughout the whole compartment volume. Such a volume may be anatomically well defined, or be a functional physiological concept. However, regardless of the nature of the compartment, the theoretical and mathematical treatment is the same. These concepts are central to any description of pharmacokinetic compartments.

MULTICOMPARTMENT MODELS - GENERAL PROPERTIES

Multicompartment pharmacokinetic models have some properties in common. These will be discussed in this section and referred to when discussing specific versions of these models.

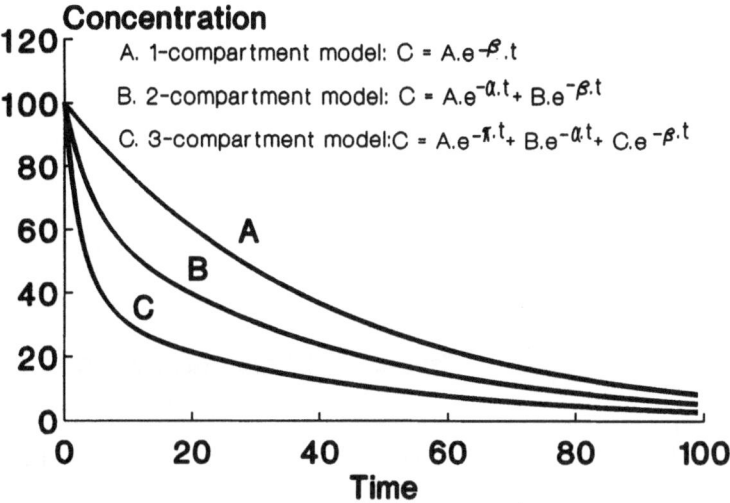

Figure 3.1: Drug concentration-time curves are shown for a drug administered by bolus intravenous injection at time = 0. The drug dose in all three curves is the same, only the curves differ because 1-, 2- and 3-compartment model equations were used to generate them.

Multi-exponential curves

Multicompartment pharmacokinetic models are based on the empirical observation that the blood drug concentration-time curve of a drug after a single rapid intravenous injection of that drug may be described by a single or a multiple exponential equation. The implication of this observation is that the drug is distributed in only one drug containing compartment for a drug whose concentration-time curve can be described by a single exponential equation. If the concentration-time curve can to be described by an equation containing two exponential terms, then the drug is distributed throughout two drug containing compartments. The number of exponential terms in the equation is identical to the number of compartments in which the drug is distributed. All anesthetic drugs have kinetics which can be described by either 2- or 3-compartment models.

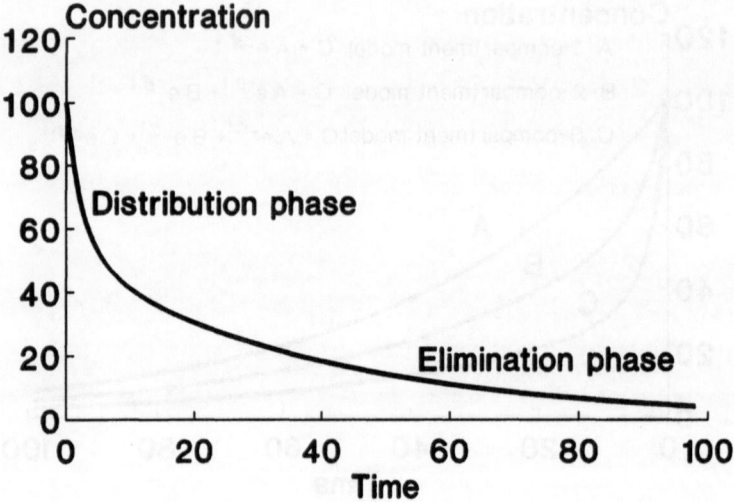

Figure 3.2: A typical concentration-time curve of a drug after a single rapid intravenous injection, where the curve can be described by a multi-exponential equation. The initial rapid decline of drug concentration is due to distribution of the drug within the body, the "distribution phase". The slower decline of plasma concentration is determined by the rate of drug elimination, and so is called the "elimination phase".

Distribution and elimination phases

The plasma concentration-time curve of a drug administered as a single rapid intravenous dose may be divided into a **distribution phase** and an **elimination phase**. These two phases are shown in figure 3.2.

Distribution phase

After a drug is administered intravenously it is initially only present in the blood, and so the concentration is high. Blood transports the drug to all the organs and tissues of the body, and the drug concentration falls rapidly due to diffusion of drug out of capillaries and venules into tissues and organs. This whole process is one where the drug is distributed throughout the body. So it is not surprising that this period is called the **distribution phase**.

Elimination phase

After drug distribution throughout all the tissues and organs of the body is complete, the only process by which the blood drug concentration can fall is by elimination of the drug from the body. Drug elimination is relatively slow in comparison to drug distribution. This means that drug elimination causes the blood concentration of a drug to decline at a slower rate than does drug distribution, and is the reason that drug concentration declines more slowly after the distribution phase has passed. The period after the distribution phase is therefore called the elimination phase, as it is drug elimination which determines the rate of decline of blood drug concentration.

The fact that the elimination phase begins after the distribution phase has passed does not mean that no drug elimination occurs during the distribution phase. This is most emphatically not the case. Drug is eliminated during the distribution phase too. However, the rate at which drug is eliminated only becomes evident after the administered drug dose has been distributed throughout the body.

Redistribution

The major proportion of the cardiac output flows to the "vessel-rich" group of tissues [see tables 2.3 and 2.4]. A consequence of this is that at any one time more drug containing blood flows through "vessel-rich" tissues than through "vessel-poor" tissues. This means that drug concentrations in the "vessel-rich" tissues can rise and fall more rapidly than in the "vessel-poor" tissues [see discussion on blood flow and drug diffusion in chapter 2]. So shortly after intravenous injection of a drug, in the beginning of the distribution phase, most of the injected drug flows to, and diffuses into the "vessel-rich" tissues. Diffusion of the injected drug into ALL tissues causes blood drug concentration to fall. When blood drug concentration falls below that in the "vessel-rich" tissues, drug diffuses out of these tissues into the blood to be distributed to other tissues with a lower blood flow. Such a shift of drug from "high-flow" to "low-flow" tissues is called **redistribution**.

Redistribution is a process that is influenced to a major degree by tissue blood flow, as it is blood which transports the drug around the body to the organs in which it is distributed. Indeed, the redistribution rate of thiopental has been found to be directly proportional to the cardiac output [6].

Central and peripheral compartments

Shortly after intravenous injection, the majority of the administered drug dose is present in blood and "vessel-rich" tissues [see above]. The "vessel-rich" tissues form a functional pharmacokinetic compartment where rapid drug exchange can occur between blood and extravascular tissues. This compartment is called the **central compartment**, or V_c. Blood or plasma volume are also part of the central compartment volume. However, blood volume is only a relatively small fraction of the central compartment volume for most drugs. Blood volume is only about 0.07 L/kg body weight, while drug central compartment volumes are usually much larger than this, [see appendix-A].

After (re-)distribution, an administered drug is distributed in both "vessel-rich" and "vessel-poor" tissues. This is the **volume of distribution** of a drug, usually written V_d. Subtraction of the central compartment volume from the distribution volume leaves a volume called the **peripheral compartment volume.**

Volume of drug distribution

If a drug is added to a volume of solvent, the concentration of that drug after it has distributed throughout that volume of solvent is given by equation 3.1.

$$\text{Concentration} = C = \frac{\text{amount}}{\text{volume}} = \frac{\text{Dose}}{V} \tag{3.1}$$

The situation often arises where the amount and the concentration of a drug are known, but the volume in which it is distributed is unknown. Rearrangement of equation 3.1 then gives the volume in which that drug is dissolved.

$$V = \frac{\text{Dose}}{C} \tag{3.2}$$

Dose is the drug dose.
V is the volume of distribution of the drug.
C is the drug concentration.

Equation 3.2 is a statement of the method currently used to determine the distribution volumes of drugs. Distribution volume of a drug is determined by serially measuring plasma or blood drug concentrations for a time after administering a known dose of the drug being investigated. Statistical procedures are then used to determine the multicompartment pharmacokinetic model best able to describe the concentration-time curve observed for that drug dose. The parameters of the chosen multicompartment model can then be used to calculate the distribution volumes of the drug being investigated.

Some factors which determine the extent of drug distribution will now be discussed.

Drugs confined to plasma volume

The volume of distribution of all drugs unable to diffuse into erythrocytes or out of blood vessels is the plasma volume. This is caused by a variety of factors.

- Capillary endothelium is relatively impermeable to molecules whose molecular weight is above 10,000 g/mole [1]. Erythrocyte membranes are also impermeable to such large molecules. This means that the volume throughout which such a substance is distributed is the plasma volume. Examples of such large molecules are the proteins and high molecular weight dextrans (MW > 70,000 g/mole).

• Drugs which are fat-insoluble do not readily diffuse into erythrocytes. If all of the drug present in plasma is also bound to proteins, as well as being eliminated rapidly, then the volume of distribution of such a drug is equal to the plasma volume. In this situation the drug does not stay in the body long enough for significant quantities of the drug to diffuse out of blood vessels. A good example of such a substance is indocyanine green, a dye used for measurement of cardiac output [see example 3.1].

EXAMPLE 3.1:

Indocyanine green is a substance which is very highly protein bound, and has a very short elimination half life which is equal to 3.8 minutes [2]. In figure 1 in a paper by Weigand et al (1960) [2], an example was given of an adult man to whom 28.54 mg of indocyanine green was administered intravenously. The initial plasma drug concentration in this man was 11 mg/L.

-    Dose = 28.54 mg.
-    Concentration = C = 11 mg/L.
-    Volume of distribution = Dose/C = 28.54/11 = 2.594 liters, a volume which is equal to the plasma volume of the average adult.

Drugs confined to the extracellular fluid volume

Capillary and venular endothelium are very permeable to molecules with a molecular weight of less than 10,000 g/mole [1]. All drugs used in anesthesia have a molecular weight which is much less than 10,000 g/mole [see appendix-B]. This means that any drug which is injected intravenously will at least distribute throughout the extracellular fluid volume. The extracellular fluid volume is the plasma volume plus the interstitial fluid volume.

A drug which is fat-insoluble and highly ionized cannot diffuse rapidly into cells in any significant quantity. So if the molecular weight of such a drug is also well below 10,000 g/mole, its distribution volume is only the extracellular fluid volume. One class of drugs fits this description very well, the non-depolarizing muscle relaxants.

EXAMPLE 3.2:

The extracellular fluid volume is about 20% of the total body weight of a normal adult. (Note: the density of a human body is nearly the same as the density of water.)

In an investigation reported by Ramzan et al (1981) [3], healthy surgical patients were administered 2 mg/kg gallamine intravenously. The resulting plasma gallamine concentration after full distribution of the administered gallamine had occurred was 9 mg/L, [see figure 1 in the paper by Ramzan et al (1960) [3]].

- Dose = 2 mg/kg.
- Concentration = C = 9 mg/L.
- Volume of distribution = Dose/C = 2/9 = 0.222 L/kg, a volume which approximates the extracellular fluid volume of a normal adult quite well.

Fat solubility

Many drugs are fat soluble to some degree. The effects of fat solubility on the distribution volume of a drug can best be illustrated using an example.

EXAMPLE 3.3:

Fentanyl is a very fat soluble drug, being 35 times more soluble in adipose tissue than in plasma [see appendix-B].

- Consider an experimental setup where a two liter container of blood is divided into two one liter compartments by a membrane permeable to fentanyl. Add 36 mg of fentanyl to one of the compartments. Allow sufficient time for the fentanyl to diffuse into the opposite compartment and the concentrations to equilibrate. Measure the fentanyl concentration in the compartment to which the fentanyl was added. The concentration will be 18 mg/L. This means that the volume of distribution is two liters, precisely what would be expected as the solvent concentration on either side of the membrane is the same.

- Now consider an experimental setup similar to that above. One half of the 2 liter container is again filled with blood, separated from the other half by a membrane permeable to fentanyl. The second half of the container is filled with adipose tissue. Add 36 mg of fentanyl to the compartment containing blood. Then wait sufficient time for the fentanyl concentrations in both compartments to equilibrate. On measuring the fentanyl concentration in the blood containing compartment it is found that the concentration of fentanyl is only 1 mg/L. This is hardly surprising as the adipose tissue/whole blood partition coefficient is 35/1, i.e. fentanyl is 35 times more soluble in adipose tissue than in whole blood. So 35 mg of the 36 mg fentanyl added to the blood compartment has diffused into, and is dissolved in the adipose tissue containing compartment. If the fentanyl concentration in the blood containing compartment is used to determine the distribution volume of the fentanyl, a surprising result is found.

    - Dose of fentanyl added to blood compartment = 36 mg.

- Fentanyl concentration measured in blood compartment = 1 mg/L.
- Therefore volume of distribution = V = Dose/C = 36/1 = 36 liters!

The volume of distribution is much greater than the total physical volume of both the compartments combined (2 liters).

Example 3.3 clearly shows that the large volumes of distribution for fat soluble drugs are a result of the method of determining the volumes of distribution by measuring plasma drug concentrations. For example, the drugs haloperidol, thiopental, fentanyl, and methadone are very fat soluble and have volumes of distribution which are very much larger than that of the human body.

Protein binding

The volume throughout which a drug is distributed is inversely proportional to the percentage of the drug present in the plasma that is bound to plasma proteins. A high percentage binding of a given drug means that very little unbound drug can diffuse out of capillaries. A good example of such a substance is indocyanine green [2]. The reverse is true for drugs which are minimally protein bound.

Degree of ionization

Drugs are chemicals which are water soluble to a greater or lesser degree, and exist in both non-ionized and ionized forms in aqueous solution.

pKa

Percentage ionization of a drug in solution is a function of the **pKa** of that drug. The pKa is the pH of the solution in which a drug is dissolved, at which 50% of the drug in solution is ionized. Water is the principal solvent in the human body, and so the pKa values mentioned in this book are for drugs in aqueous solution. Appendix-B lists pKa values of many drugs used in anesthetic practice.

Degree of ionization

Drugs behave as either acids or bases in aqueous solution. Degree of ionization of a drug is determined by the pH of the solution, and whether a drug is an acid or a base.

- The percentage ionization of acidic drugs increases if the pH of the solution increases, and decreases if the solution pH decreases.

- Percentage ionization of basic drugs decreases as the solution pH increases, and increases as the pH of the solution decreases.

Because a drug may behave as either an acid or a base, two different equations are required to calculate the percentage ionization of drugs in solution [equations 3.3 and 3.4].

$$\% \text{Ionization(acids)} = 100 \times \frac{10^{(pH - pKa)}}{1 + 10^{(pH - pKa)}} \qquad (3.3)$$

$$\% \text{Ionization(bases)} = 100 \times \frac{10^{(pKa - pH)}}{1 + 10^{(pKa - pH)}} \qquad (3.4)$$

pH is the pH of the fluid in which a drug is dissolved.
pKa is pH of the solution at which a drug is 50% ionized.

Ionization and fat-solubility

Ionized molecules or atoms are not fat-soluble. Such atoms or molecules cannot easily diffuse through lipid cell membranes. However ionized substances can enter cells if they are transported through the cell membrane through special channels, e.g. calcium and sodium channels. The same applies to drugs. A drug cannot rapidly diffuse through cell membranes unless it is fat-soluble and non-ionized.

"Ion-trapping"

The situation frequently arises in the body where there is a lipid membrane with a solution on either side whose pH is different. For example, the plasma has a pH of 7.4. However intracellular pH is somewhat lower, ranging from 7.3 down to 6.5 [4]. In fact a pH gradient exists between nearly all fluid containing compartments of the body.

Diffusion of the non-ionized form of a drug causes the concentrations of the non-ionized form of a given drug to eventually equalize on either side of a lipid membrane. However the total drug concentrations may be different on each side because the drug is more ionized on one side than the other. Such a situation arises because the ionized form of the drug cannot diffuse through the membrane. This phenomenon is called "ion-trapping".

The relative concentrations of an ionizable drug in two solutions of differing pH separated by a lipid membrane, where the protein binding and fat solubility on either side are equal are given by equations 3.5 and 3.6 [1, page 30].

$$\text{ACIDS} = \frac{C_1}{C_2} = \frac{1 + 10^{(pH1 - pKa)}}{1 + 10^{(pH2 - pKa)}} \qquad (3.5)$$

$$\text{BASES} = \frac{C_1}{C_2} = \frac{1 + 10^{(pKa - pH1)}}{1 + 10^{(pKa - pH2)}} \qquad (3.6)$$

pH_1, pH_2 is the pH of the solutions in compartments 1 and 2 respectively.
C_1, C_2 are the drug concentrations in compartments 1 and 2 respectively.

EXAMPLE 3.4:

Consider the drug fentanyl, and the effect of ion-trapping on concentration differences between fentanyl in plasma, cerebrospinal fluid (CSF), and gastric fluid.

The pKa of fentanyl = 8.4, and fentanyl is a base. Therefore use equation 3.6.

Plasma - CSF difference

Plasma pH = 7.4; Percentage fentanyl ionization = 90.71%
CSF pH = 7.35; Percentage fentanyl ionization = 91.8%

Let CSF be compartment 1, and plasma be compartment 2. Equation 3.6 can be used to show that C_1/C_2 = 1.11. Fentanyl concentration in the CSF is 11% higher than in plasma.

Plasma - Gastric fluid difference

Plasma pH = 7.4; Percentage fentanyl ionization = 90.71%
Gastric pH = 3.0; Percentage fentanyl ionization = 99.7999%

Let the gastric fluid be compartment 1 and plasma be compartment 2. Equation 3.6 shows that C_1/C_2 = 22835, meaning that the predicted gastric fluid fentanyl concentration is 22835 times higher than that in plasma! The gastric fluid/plasma fentanyl concentration ratio has been measured in human subjects undergoing surgery and has actually been found to be about 200 instead of 22835 [5]. This is much less than predicted. However 84% of fentanyl in plasma is bound to plasma proteins, reducing the amount of fentanyl available for diffusion into the stomach. This accounts for part of the discrepancy between the predicted and measured concentration ratio.

A high gastric fluid fentanyl concentration may cause postoperative respiratory depression in persons who have received fentanyl during surgery. This is especially likely if the gastric fluid volume is considerable. In this situation intestinal absorption of significant amounts of fentanyl may occur. This may be one of the causes of the delayed postoperative respiratory depression occasionally reported after use of fentanyl [5].

Clearance

Clearance is a concept which is extensively used in pharmacokinetics, especially when considering intravenous infusions. Unfortunately it is a concept which is sometimes difficult to understand for the student beginning to learn pharmacokinetics. So it will be discussed in some detail.

Drug elimination

It is useful to define drug elimination. **Elimination** of a drug is the removal of that drug from the blood or body by metabolism, excretion or both. The **elimination rate** is the amount of drug which is removed from the body or blood per unit time.

The elimination rate constant

A basic property of a pharmacokinetic compartment is that the concentration of drug throughout the volume of the compartment is always the same. The volume of drug containing fluid removed from a pharmacokinetic compartment per unit time is also constant. A consequence of this is that a constant fraction of the total amount of the drug contained within the compartment is removed per unit time. This constant fraction of the total volume of drug containing fluid in the compartment that is removed per unit time is expressed as a rate constant, k_{el}, the **elimination rate constant** [see figure 3.3]. The unit used is time^{-1}.

Figure 3.3: The rate constant of drug exit from the 1-compartment model of figure 1.4 has been changed to the more usual term, "k_{el}" which denotes "elimination rate constant".

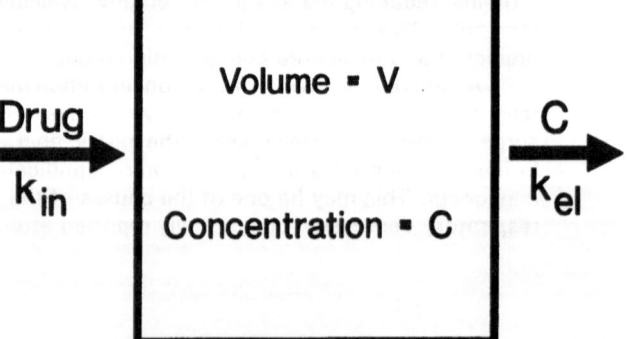

Clearance

If the volume of the pharmacokinetic compartment from which a drug is eliminated is multiplied by the k_{el} for that drug, the product is the volume of drug containing fluid in that compartment which is eliminated from that compartment per unit time. This is the **drug clearance**.

$$Cl = V.k_{el} \qquad (3.7)$$

V is the volume of the pharmacokinetic compartment.
Cl is the drug clearance.

Clearance of any given drug is a constant which is different for each drug. It is not related to the concentration of that drug, because drug concentration is not a factor which determines clearance. Only two factors define drug clearance from a compartment, k_{el} and V, and these are constants. The units by which clearance is expressed are volume/time. This may be confirmed by dimensional analysis.

The usual units used to express clearance in current pharmacokinetic literature are **ml/kg body weight/minute**. These units are not used in this book. Instead clearance is expressed as **liters/kg body weight/hour**. The reason for this is simple. It makes calculating drug infusion rates much easier.

Elimination rate

Multiplying drug clearance by the concentration of the drug in the pharmacokinetic compartment at that time gives the amount of drug eliminated from the compartment per unit time. This is the **elimination rate**.

$$Q_{el} = C.Cl \qquad (3.8)$$

C is the drug concentration at that time.
Q_{el} is the amount of drug eliminated per unit time, i.e. the **elimination rate**.
Cl is the drug clearance as volume/time.

EXAMPLE 3.5:

Consider an adult to whom a 10 mg dose of morphine has been administered intravenously. When the drug is fully distributed throughout the body, (a process that actually takes about 20 minutes but which for the sake of this example will be considered to be instantaneous), the plasma morphine concentration is about 0.028 mg/L.

The whole body clearance of morphine is 2 L/kg/h, i.e. about 140 L/h for an average 70 kg adult. A clearance of 140 L/h means that shortly after intravenous morphine administration that the elimination rate of morphine = Q_{el} = C.Cl = 0.028 x 140 = 3.72 mg/h.

After 1 elimination half life the plasma morphine concentration has declined to 0.014 mg/L. At this time the elimination rate of morphine = Q_{el} = C.Cl = 0.014 x 140 = 1.76 mg/h.

In other words, drug elimination rate is related to the concentration of the drug in the compartment from which it is being eliminated, but clearance is a constant factor which is quite independent of the drug concentration.

Various methods of expressing drug clearance

There are several ways of expressing drug clearance.

Plasma clearance

Here the concentration of the drug concerned is the plasma drug concentration. Plasma clearance is a measure of the rate at which a drug is cleared from plasma.

Blood clearance

Here the drug concentration concerned is the whole blood drug concentration. Blood clearance is a measure of clearance of drug from whole blood. This is the clearance which should be used when considering individual organ clearance of a drug. The reason for this is that when drug containing blood passes through an organ, not only drug contained in the plasma enters that organ, but drug also diffuses out of erythrocytes into plasma. This increases the amount of drug in plasma which is available for diffusion into organs or tissues.

Intrinsic organ clearance

This is the clearance of a drug by a specific organ. For example, **renal clearance** is the clearance of drug by the kidneys alone, and **hepatic clearance** is the clearance of a drug by the liver alone.

Extraction ratio

Extraction ratio is a concept which is related to intrinsic organ clearance. It is defined by equations 3.9 and 3.10.

$$\text{Clearance} = \text{Organ Blood Flow} \times \text{Extraction ratio} \qquad (3.9)$$

or

$$Cl = Q \times \frac{(C_a - C_v)}{C_a} \qquad (3.10)$$

C_a is the arterial whole blood drug concentration.
C_v is the venous whole blood drug concentration.
$(C_a - C_v)/C_a$ is the extraction ratio.
Q is the organ blood flow.

For any given organ the extraction ratio of a particular drug may be either "high" or "low". This has several consequences for the kinetics of a given drug.

Low extraction ratio drugs

There are several reasons why a given drug has a low extraction ratio.

- The drug may diffuse very slowly out of the blood into the organ where the extraction ratio is low.

- It may be removed from the blood by a saturable transport system.

- The drug may be excreted or metabolized by the organ very slowly.

In the case of low extration ratio drugs, blood flow is usually able to deliver more drug per unit time than can be extracted by organs extracting those drugs, even when flow is low. In other words, removal of low extraction ratio drugs from the blood is not dependant on organ blood flow.

High extraction ratio drugs

High extraction ratio drugs are those whose rate of extraction from blood is not limited by saturable excretory, metabolic, or transport systems. Clearance of such drugs is not limited by the rate at which the organ eliminates the drug, but by the rate at which drug is transported to the eliminating organ. In this situation drug extraction is limited by the organ blood flow or cardiac output. A drug which has a high extraction ratio, and which is eliminated solely by a particular organ, has a clearance which is nearly equal to the blood flow to the eliminating organ.

1-COMPARTMENT MODEL

Because of the physiology and anatomy of the body, all drugs must first undergo a distribution phase. So a 1-compartment model is by definition unable to adequately describe the kinetics of any drug. This does not mean that the 1-compartment pharmacokinetic model is only an academic curiosity. In fact the 1-compartment pharmacokinetic model is of considerable practical and didactic utility.

- One situation in which this model can be applied is to drug containing compartments where there is **only one** source of drug input into a compartment, and **only one** source of drug loss from that compartment. This means that such a model applies to drug kinetics in individual organs such as the heart chambers, fat tissue, liver etc. Such a use of this model is described in chapters 1 and 2.

- A 1-compartment pharmacokinetic model is capable of providing insights into the basic properties of multicompartment kinetic models. This application has already been demonstrated in chapters 1 and 2.

- Single-compartment drug kinetics can be used to simplify calculations where a multicompartment kinetic model is used. The distribution and elimination phases of a multicompartment model can be considered separately using a 1-compartment model to describe each phase. This application is demonstrated in chapter 5, and used extensively in other chapters.

1-Compartment Model

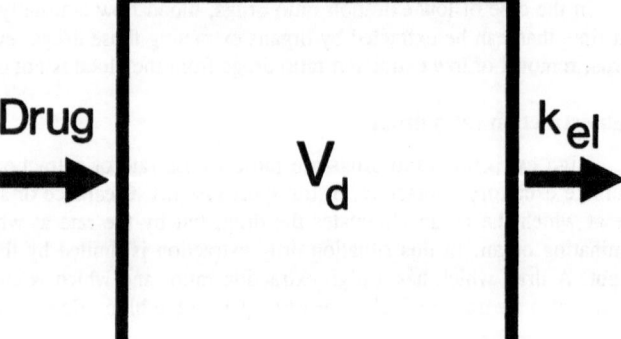

Figure 3.4: The elements of the 1-compartment model are shown. There is a single compartment into which a drug can enter, and from which it can leave.

Single drug dose and the 1-compartment model

After administration of a drug dose into a single kinetic compartment, the drug mixes instantly throughout the compartment volume. Drug elimination then causes the concentration of that drug to decline exponentially in the manner shown in figure 3.5. The change of drug concentration with time may be described with either a differential or an exponential equation [equations 3.11 and 3.12 respectively].

Differential equation [see chapter 1 for method of derivation]

$$\frac{dC}{dt} = -C.k_{el} \tag{3.11}$$

Exponential equation

$$C_t = A.e^{-\beta t} \tag{3.12}$$

t is the elapsed time after drug injection.
C_t is the concentration of drug at any given time "t".
A is the initial plasma drug concentration at the instant of injection.
β is the fraction of drug eliminated per unit time and $= k_{el}$ in the 1-compartment model.

Figure 3.5: Plasma concentration-time curve resulting from administration of a single intravenous dose of a drug whose kinetics can be described by a 1-compartment model.

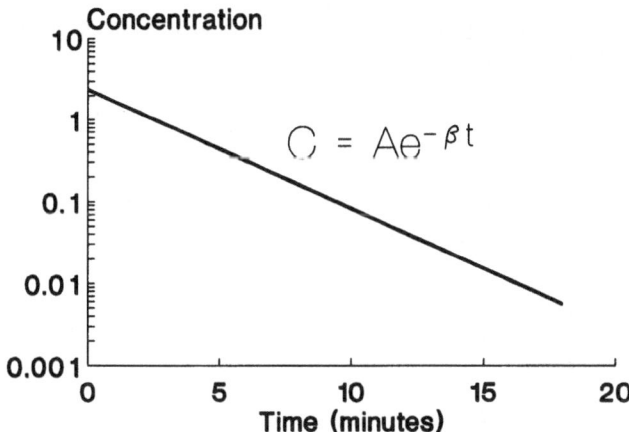

Distribution volume

In the 1-compartment model there is only one compartment throughout which the drug is distributed. This is called the distribution volume and is designated V_d.

Measurement of the V_d is not so easy. One problem with a living organism is that an administered drug is continually eliminated from the body. So the plasma concentration continually falls. This means that V_d cannot simply be estimated from a single measurement of the plasma drug concentration. The method used to surmount this problem is to use the plasma concentration-time curve after drug administration to derive the kinetic parameters A and β in equation 3.12. These derived values may be substituted into equation 3.12, and time set at "0" seconds. The value of C_t

is then calculated. This is assumed to be the drug concentration existing in the distribution volume immediately after drug administration, when no drug elimination has occurred. So at t = 0 seconds, equation 3.12 becomes equation 3.13.

$$C_0 = A = \frac{\text{Dose}}{V_d} \qquad (3.13)$$

Elimination constant

A constant fraction of the drug present in the V_d is eliminated per unit time. This is the reason for the exponential decay curve. The elimination constant is usually designated as $\mathbf{k_{el}}$ in the multicompartment models. In the 1-compartment model this elimination constant may also be designated with the greek letter β. This has precisely the same meaning.

Elimination half life ($t_{1/2\beta}$)

The only half life to be considered in the 1-compartment model is the elimination half life. This is usually designated "$t_{1/2\beta}$". It is related to the elimination rate constant in the manner shown by equation 3.14.

$$t_{1/2\beta} = \frac{0.693}{k_{el}} = \frac{0.693}{\beta} \qquad (3.14)$$

The relationship of plasma drug concentration to the elimination half life for a monoexponential equation is shown in table 3.1.

Clearance (Cl)

Clearance has been discussed earlier in this chapter. It is related to the V_d and $t_{1/2\beta}$ as is shown below.

Equation 3.7 gives the clearance of a drug in a 1-compartment system.

$$Cl = V_d \cdot k_{el} \qquad (3.7)$$

Now $t_{1/2\beta}$ is related to k_{el} by equation 3.14.

$$t_{1/2\beta} = \frac{0.693}{k_{el}} \qquad (3.14)$$

Rearrangement, and substitution of equation 3.14 into 3.7 yields a relationship showing how these three factors are interrelated.

$$t_{1/2\beta} = \frac{0.693 \times V_d}{Cl} \qquad (3.15)$$

Table 3.1.

Relationship between the multiple of the elimination half life of a drug and its plasma concentration for a **1-compartment model**. Two situations are shown, increasing and decreasing drug concentrations. An example of an **exponentially increasing** drug concentration is the drug concentration-time curve due to a constant rate intravenous infusion. The concentration-time curve resulting from a single rapid intravenous dose of a drug is a good example of an **exponentially decreasing** concentration.

Multiple of elimination half life	INCREASING CONCN. Plasma drug concn. as % of TARGET concn. (original concn. = 0 and target = 100)	DECREASING CONCN. Plasma drug concn. as % of ORIGINAL concn. (original concn. = 100 and target = 0)
0	0	100
1	50	50
2	75	25
3	87.5	12.5
4	93.75	6.25
5	96.875	3.125

Limitations of the 1-compartment model

Despite the many didactic and practical advantages, the reader should not lose sight of the fact that the 1-compartment model is inadequate to describe the kinetics of intravenously injected drugs. The reason for this is simply due to the physiological and anatomical structure of the body. There are "vessel-rich" and "vessel-poor" tissues. The majority of an intravenously injected dose of a drug is always distributed to "vessel-rich" organs first, after which (re)distribution to "vessel-poor" tissues also occurs. Accordingly a multicompartment pharmacokinetic model is always required to describe the kinetics of intravenously administered drugs.

2-COMPARTMENT MODEL

The simplest multicompartment model is the 2-compartment model. This is fortunately a model which is also clinically relevant and provides a reasonably accurate description of the behavior of most drugs used in anesthetic practice.

Basic elements of the 2-compartment model

The 2-compartment pharmacokinetic model assumes that an administered drug is at first distributed within a central compartment, usually designated V_c or V_1. Drug is subsequently eliminated from V_1, and exchanged between V_1 and a **peripheral** or **deep** drug compartment designated V_2. The fractional rate of transfer, (rate constant), of drug from V_1 to V_2 is given by the constant k_{12}, and the fractional rate of transfer of drug from V_2 to V_1 is given by k_{21}. The conceptual elements of this model are shown in figure 3.6.

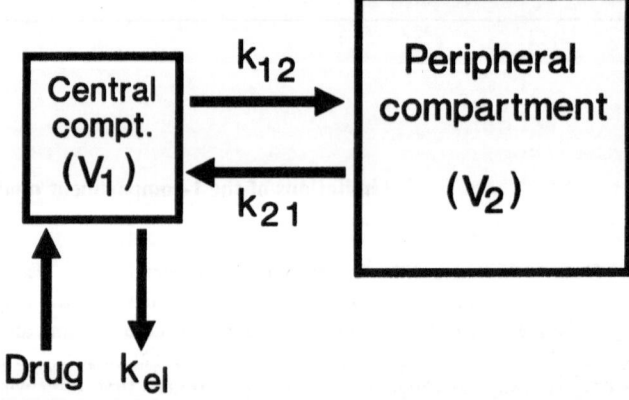

Figure 3.6: Conceptual elements of the 2-compartment pharmacokinetic model.

Single intravenous dose

Many drugs used in clinical anesthetic practice have kinetics able to be described by a 2-compartment model. When a single dose of a drug is administered intravenously over a very short period of time, the drug is initially only present in V_1. The drug diffuses into V_2, and at the same time drug is also eliminated from V_1. Drug continues to diffuse into V_2 until the drug concentration in V_1 falls below that in V_2. After this drug concentration in V_1 falls due to drug elimination, and drug concentration in V_2 falls due to diffusion of drug into V_1. This situation is depicted in figure 3.7.

The basic equations describing drug concentrations in V_1 and V_2 for the situation where a drug is injected rapidly into V_1 are given below in both their differential and exact forms. The differential equations have already been derived in chapter 1 using the techniques explained there [see figure 1.5b and equations 1.20 and 1.21].

Differential equations

$$\frac{dC_1}{dt} = C_2.k_{21} - C_1.k_{el} - C_1.k_{12} \tag{3.16}$$

$$\frac{dC_2}{dt} = C_1.k_{12} - C_2.k_{21} \tag{3.17}$$

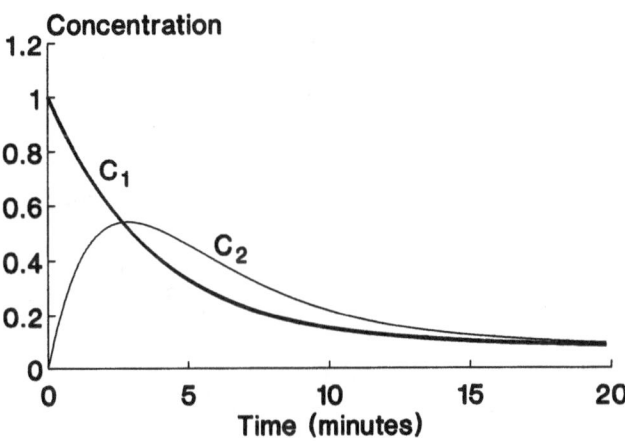

Figure 3.7: Central (C_1) and peripheral (C_2) compartment drug concentrations resulting from a single intravenous dose of a drug whose kinetics can be described by a 2-compartment model. Note that the central compartment drug concentration is the same as that in the plasma, as plasma is part of the central compartment.

Exact solutions of the equations 3.16 and 3.17

$$C_1 = A.e^{-\alpha t} + B.e^{-\beta t} \tag{3.18}$$

$$C_2 = L.e^{-\alpha t} + M.e^{-\beta t} \tag{3.19}$$

C_1 and C_2 are the drug concentrations in V_1 and V_2 respectively. C_1 is also the plasma drug concentration.

B is a term giving the plasma concentration of a drug were it to be fully distributed throughout its' whole distribution volume the instant after intravenous injection. This a purely hypothetical situation, and so is an extrapolated value.

A is a term which when added to **B** gives the plasma or blood drug concentration the instant after intravenous injection of a single drug dose. This term corrects for the fact that the initial volume of drug distribution, (equal to the central compartment volume), is much smaller than the whole volume of distribution of a drug [see figure 3.5].

L and **M** are terms analogous to **A** and **B** respectively, only they describe drug concentrations in the peripheral drug compartment [see figure 3.5].

α is a constant describing the rate of (re)distribution of a drug from V_1 to the whole drug distribution volume.

β is a constant describing the rate of drug elimination from the body.

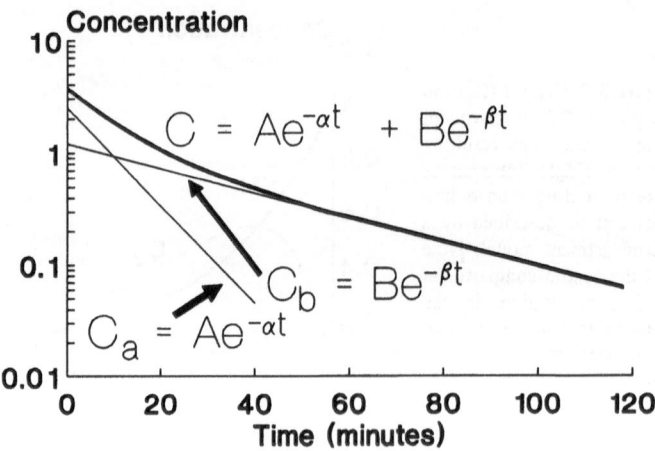

Figure 3.8: The plasma concentration in the 2-compartment kinetic model is the sum of the concentrations given by the sum of the two mon-oexponential components of the model.

When $t = 0$ in equation 3.18, both exponents $= 0$. Now $e^0 = 1$, and so equation 3.18 reduces to equation 3.20 which gives the theoretical plasma drug concentration at the instant that the rapid intravenous administration of a drug is complete.

$$\text{at } t = 0, \text{ then } C_0 = A + B \tag{3.20}$$

Half lives

The constants α and β are used to describe the rates of distribution and elimination. These processes also have half lives described by equations 3.21 and 3.22 below [see equation 1.10 in chapter 1 for derivation of half lives].

$$\text{Distribution half life} = t_{1/2\alpha} = \frac{0.693}{\alpha} \tag{3.21}$$

$$\text{Elimination half life} = t_{1/2\beta} = \frac{0.693}{\beta} \tag{3.22}$$

Determination of Central Compartment volume

The volume of V_1 or V_c can be calculated by dividing the total dose of a drug by the theoretical drug concentration existing the instant after drug administration. The theoretical concentration at the instant that drug administration is complete given by equation 3.20. As the drug dose is known, the volume of V_1 can be calculated using equation 3.23 below.

$$V_1 = V_c = \frac{\text{Dose}}{A + B} \tag{3.23}$$

Distribution volumes (V_d, V_{ss}, V_{ext}, V_{area}, V_β)

There are various definitions of distribution volume in the 2-compartment kinetic model. A general term for the distribution volume is "V_d". However this says nothing about which distribution volume is referred to in any specific case. So when viewing the kinetic data of a drug one should always carefully ascertain the distribution volume used or presented. The various distribution volumes in common use are defined below.

Steady state volume of distribution (V_{ss})

If a drug is administered at a constant rate for a long time, the concentration of that drug in V_2 will eventually equal the concentration in V_1. Drug concentration in both compartments is in equilibrium. This condition is called **steady state**.

Such a condition is only possible if the rate of transfer of drug from V_1 to V_2 equals that from V_2 to V_1 as described by equation 3.24.

$$V_1 . k_{12} = V_2 . k_{21} \tag{3.24}$$

Under the conditions as defined by equation 3.24 the volume of distribution will therefore be defined by equation 3.25. This is the steady state volume of distribution and is usually designated by V_{ss}.

$$V_{ss} = V_1 + V_2 \tag{3.25}$$

However there is a major limitation to the use of the V_{ss} in practical clinical situations. The main problem is that the V_{ss} is a volume of distribution which is defined for steady state conditions. Such conditions are only present during intravenous infusions which have been administered for a very long time. This situation never occurs when drugs are administered as intermittent intravenous boluses. Therefore any use of this distribution volume for calculations performed under non-steady state conditions is incorrect.

Extrapolated volume of distribution (V_{ext})

After a single rapid intravenous injection of a drug dose, the change of plasma drug concentration with time is given by equation 3.18. Once drug (re-)distribution is complete, change of drug concentration with time is given by $C = Be^{-\beta t}$ alone as the term $Ae^{-\alpha t} = 0$. If the concentration given by this monoexponential term is extrapolated back to zero time, then $C = B$, as $e^{-\beta t} = 1$ at this time. This means that the extrapolated volume of distribution (V_{ext}) can be defined by equation 3.26 [reference 7, equations 2-124 and 2-125].

$$V_{ext} = \frac{Dose}{B} = \frac{V_1(\alpha - \beta)}{(k_{21} - \beta)} \tag{3.26}$$

This is a useful definition of the distribution volume as it assumes a constantly changing plasma drug concentration.

Non steady-state volume of distribution (V_{area} and V_β)

After a single intravenous injection of a drug, the volume throughout which the drug is distributed can be related to the amount of drug present in the body as is shown by the area under the plasma drug concentration-time curve during the elimination phase. This volume of distribution is called the V_{area}. Because it defines the volume of distribution during the elimination phase, which is also known as the β-phase, it is also called V_β. Both V_β and V_{area} are equivalent and are defined by equation 3.27 [see equation 2-123, page 83, reference 7].

$$V_{area} = V_\beta = \frac{V_1 . k_{el}}{\beta} = \frac{Cl}{\beta} \tag{3.27}$$

The volume of distribution defined by equation 3.27 is frequently used in pharmacokinetic calculations.

Relationship between the various distribution volumes

The volumes of distribution represented by V_{ss}, V_{ext} and V_β are defined differently, and so they are **NOT** equivalent. They are related in the manner shown below.

$$V_{ext} > V_\beta = V_{area} > V_{ss}$$

Therefore the reader should always ascertain which volume of distribution is referred to when reading a description of the pharmacokinetics of any given drug. Unless otherwise stated the volume of distribution, V_d referred to in this book always refers to the V_{area}.

Drug clearance

Drug clearance in the 2-compartment model is defined in precisely the same way as for the 1-compartment model. Clearance is also related to both the V_β or V_{area} and β in the manner shown by equation 3.27. The last part of equation 3.27 is most interesting as it also shows the relationship between the elimination half life, volume of distribution and the clearance. It was stated earlier in this section that V_{area} was identical to V_β. Substitute equation 3.22 into equation 3.27, rearrange, and the result is equation 3.28. This is an important equation as it shows the relationship between the two basic kinetic parameters, volume of distribution and clearance.

$$t_{1/2\beta} = \frac{0.693 \times V_\beta}{Cl} \qquad (3.28)$$

NOTE that the volume of distribution referred to by equation 3.28 is the V_{area} or V_β. This equation is invalid if any other distribution volume is used.

Calculation of A and B for single intravenous doses

The above discussion is all very interesting, but regrettably has very little practical utility because tables of pharmacokinetic parameters never list the terms "A" and "B", as their magnitude depends on drug dose. They can however be calculated for any given drug dose using the series of equations listed below [reference 7, page 83].

$$\alpha = \frac{0.693}{t_{1/2\alpha}} \qquad (3.29)$$

$$\beta = \frac{0.693}{t_{1/2\beta}} \qquad (3.30)$$

$$k_{el} = \frac{Cl}{V_1} \qquad (3.31)$$

$$k_{21} = \frac{\alpha.\beta}{k_{el}} \qquad (3.32)$$

$$k_{12} = \alpha + \beta - k_{el} - k_{21} \qquad (3.33)$$

$$A = \frac{Dose(\alpha - k_{21})}{V_1(\alpha - \beta)} \tag{3.34}$$

$$B = \frac{Dose(k_{21} - \beta)}{V_1(\alpha - \beta)} \tag{3.35}$$

Now this is a rather daunting set of equations to work through if one only wishes to calculate "A" and "B". Fortunately there is a way in which this can be simplified. Inspection of the formulae for calculating "A" and "B" reveals that except for the "Dose" term, all the other terms are quite independent of the drug dose. Accordingly the author has found that "A" and "B" may be easily calculated by splitting equations 3.34 and 3.35 in the following manner.

$$A = Dose \times A_x \tag{3.36}$$

where;

$$A_x = \frac{(\alpha - k_{21})}{V_1(\alpha - \beta)} \tag{3.37}$$

and;

$$B = Dose \times B_x \tag{3.38}$$

where;

$$B_x = \frac{(k_{21} - \beta)}{V_1(\alpha - \beta)} \tag{3.39}$$

This provides two new pharmacokinetic parameters, A_x and B_x. These simplify the calculation of A and B enormously. All that is required to calculate A and B is to multiply the drug dose by A_x and B_x respectively.

Conversely, equations 3.36 and 3.38 may be used to calculate A_x and B_x from experimentally determined values of A and B for a given drug dose.

The parameters A_x and B_x have been calculated for the most commonly used anesthetic drugs and listed in appendix-A.

EXAMPLE 3.6:

A patient is administered a single intravenous bolus dose of 0.1 mg/kg pancuronium. What is the formula for calculating the plasma pancuronium concentration at any time after administration of this dose?

This requires the use of equation 3.18. The terms α, β, B_x and A_x for pancuronium are listed in appendix-A. A and B can be calculated using equations 3.36 and 3.38.

- Dose = 0.1 mg/kg.
- $\alpha = 0.0648$ min^{-1}.

-     β = 0.0061 min^{-1}.
-     A_x = 5.54 kg/L and so A = Dose x A_x = 0.1 x 5.54 = 0.554 mg/L.
-     B_x = 2.8 kg/L and so B = Dose x B_x = 0.1 x 2.8 = 0.28 mg/L.

Equation 3.18 is;

$$C = A.e^{-\alpha t} + B.e^{-\beta t}$$

Substitution of the parameters calculated above yields the formula giving the plasma pancuronium concentration in mg/L for any time after drug administration, where time is in minutes.

$$C = 0.554e^{-0.0648t} + 0.28e^{-0.0061t}$$

Application of A_x and B_x to single I.V. dose kinetics

Equation 3.18 is used to describe the plasma drug concentration-time curve resulting from administration of a single intravenous dose of a drug. The definitions of A_x and B_x can be used to modify this equation.

$$C = Ae^{-\alpha t} + Be^{-\beta t} \qquad (3.18)$$

Substitute equations 3.36 and 3.38 into equation 3.18, and rearrange to form equation 3.40.

$$C = Dose(A_x.e^{-\alpha t} + B_x.e^{-\beta t}) \qquad (3.40)$$

Equation 3.40 offers the possibility of readily calculating the intravenous dose of a drug so that a given plasma concentration of that drug is present at any given time. This is done by rearranging equation 3.40 to the form below.

$$Dose = \frac{C}{A_x.e^{-\alpha t} + B_x.e^{-\beta t}} \qquad (3.41)$$

For the special condition where the drug dose must be calculated to provide a given drug concentration at t = 0 minutes, equation 3.41 reduces to equation 3.42 as e^{-0} = 1.

$$Dose = \frac{C}{A_x + B_x} \qquad (3.42)$$

Simplified method of calculation

A method has been presented by means of which A and B can be simply calculated. This removes one of the obstacles to the routine use of equation 3.18. However calculations with equation 3.18 are arithmetically difficult. A book of mathematical tables, or an electronic calculator is always required. One of the main causes of arithmetical difficulty is due to the base of the exponential terms. The author has found that changing the base of these exponential terms to two, together with the application of a few simple rules, greatly simplifies calculations, as well as providing formulae of considerable clinical and didactic utility.

Consider equation 3.18;

$$C = Ae^{-\alpha t} + Be^{-\beta t} \qquad (3.18)$$

Let;

$$n = \frac{t}{t_{1/2\alpha}} \qquad (3.43)$$

So;

$$\alpha t = \frac{0.693t}{t_{1/2\alpha}} = 0.693n$$

Let;

$$N = \frac{t}{t_{1/2\beta}} \qquad (3.44)$$

So;

$$\beta t = \frac{0.693t}{t_{1/2\beta}} = 0.693N$$

Now as $e^{-0.693} = 1/2$, this means that equation 3.18 may be restated as equation 3.45.

$$C = \frac{A}{2^n} + \frac{B}{2^N} \qquad (3.45)$$

When $N < 0.1$ then the term 2^N in equation 3.45 is nearly equal to one. Equation 3.45 can then be reduced to equation 3.46.

$$C = \frac{A}{2^n} + B \qquad (3.46)$$

Equation 3.46 is useful for roughly calculating plasma drug concentrations in the distribution phase of the plasma concentration-time curve.

Drug distribution is nearly complete after $4 \times t_{1/2\alpha}$. When the elapsed time $\geq 4 \times t_{1/2\alpha}$, then $2^n \geq 16$, and the term $A/2^n$ in equation 3.45 becomes relatively insignificant. So during the elimination phase of drug kinetics, equation 3.45 can be simplified to equation 3.47.

$$C = \frac{B}{2^N} \qquad (3.47)$$

The application of these equations to everyday clinical use of anesthetic drugs is extensively demonstrated in chapter 5.

3-COMPARTMENT MODEL

The plasma kinetics of some drugs are best described by a 3-compartment model. There are various versions of the three compartment model possible, but the one most commonly used is shown in figure 3.9.

The basic principles of this model are the same as for the 2-compartment model, except that the "fast" central compartment into which drug is administered connects to two compartments, an "intermediate" and a "slow" compartment. An extra rate constant "π" is used for the very fast rate, "α" for the intermediate compartment rate constant, and "β" for the elimination rate constant as before. The analysis and description of the behavior of the three compartment model is an extension of that required for the 2-compartment model.

3-Compartment Model

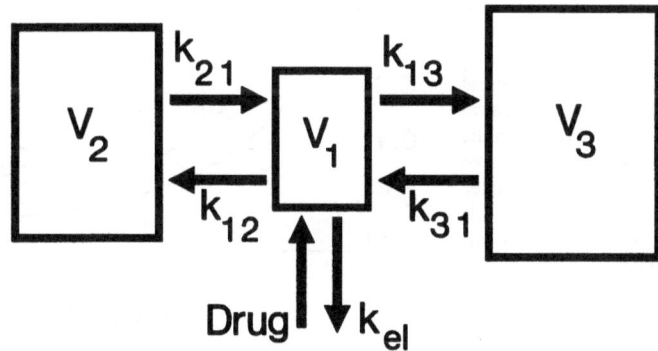

Figure 3.9: Conceptual elements of the 3-compartment pharmacokinetic model.

Single intravenous dose

After administration of a single intravenous dose of a drug it is initially only present in V_1. The drug diffuses into both V_2 and V_3, elevating the drug concentrations in both of these compartments. At the same time the drug is also eliminated from V_1. When the drug concentration in V_1

becomes lower than that in V_2 and V_3, drug concentrations in all compartments decline due to drug elimination from V_1 together with diffusion of drug from V_2 and V_3 into V_1, [see figure 3.10].

Differential equations for 3-compartment model

The series of differential equations below describes the plasma concentration of a drug after it has been rapidly administered as a single intravenous dose. Chapter 1 describes the principles which can be used to derive these equations.

$$\frac{dC_1}{dt} = C_2.k_{21} + C_3.k_{31} - C_1.k_{12} - C_1.k_{13} - C_1.k_{el} \tag{3.48}$$

$$\frac{dC_2}{dt} = C_1.k_{12} - C_2.k_{21} \tag{3.49}$$

$$\frac{dC_3}{dt} = C_1.k_{13} - C_3.k_{31} \tag{3.50}$$

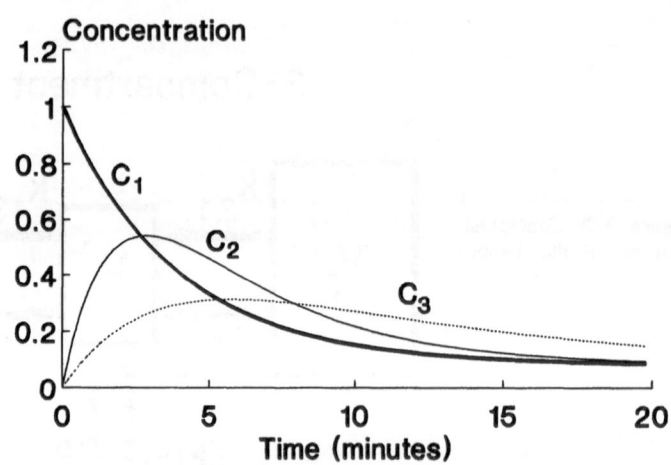

Figure 3.10: Drug concentration-time curves in the three kinetic compartments after administration of a single intravenous dose of a drug. C_1 is the plasma and central compartment concentration-time curve. C_2 is the concentration-time curve in the "intermediate" compartment, while C_3 is that of the "slow" compartment.

Exact solution of differential equation

Equation 3.51 is the exact solution of equation 3.48 and describes the plasma concentration of a drug after a single rapidly administered intravenous dose of a drug.

$$C_1 = Ae^{-\pi t} + Be^{-\alpha t} + Ce^{-\beta t} \tag{3.51}$$

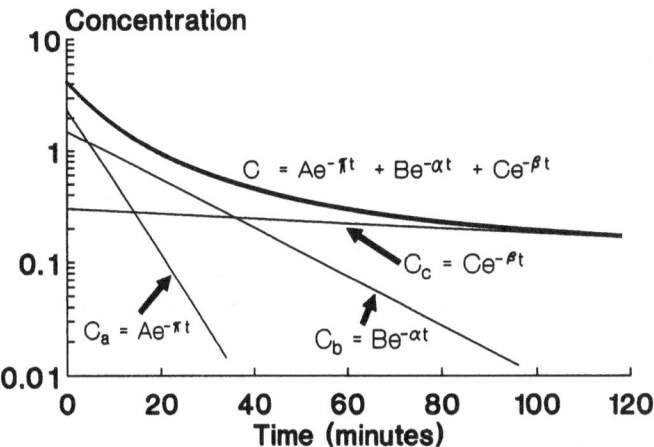

Figure 3.11: The plasma, or central compartment, concentration-time curve in the 3-compartment pharmacokinetic model is the sum of the concentrations given by each of the three monoexponential components of the model.

LIMITATIONS OF MULTI-COMPARTMENT MODELS

Mixing of a drug with the whole blood volume, or the pharmacokinetic central compartment volume after intravenous injection is not instantaneous. Some time is required for any injected drug to mix with these volumes. However all multicompartment pharmacokinetic models assume that such mixing is instantaneous, and so are totally inaccurate in their estimation of the blood concentration of a drug during the pre-recirculation phase of drug kinetics. For this reason the period immediately after intravenous injection of a drug should always be considered separately from any subsequent multicompartment analysis of drug distribution.

Recirculation of blood from the upper half of the body terminates the pre-recirculation phase 20-30 seconds after intravenous drug injection, [see chapter 2]. So the heart-lung model of chapter 2 should be used to describe the blood drug concentrations in the first 30 seconds after drug injection. A multicompartment model can used for all times subsequent to this.

VARIABILITY OF PHARMACOKINETIC PARAMETERS

The mathematical pharmacokinetic models discussed in the previous pages are very beautiful. They are capable of describing the plasma concentration of drugs at any time after administration. However, as with any mathematical model, the accuracy of any prediction is directly related to the accuracy of the data used.

The individual persons making up a population group differ considerably from one another. Some are young and others are old. There are males and females, and some of the females are pregnant. In any particular group of persons body weight varies considerably, and some persons may be unfortunate enough to have concurrent diseases. Circadian rhythms, drugs, anesthesia, and mental state also alter the physiology of the body in any one person too.

The result of all these interpersonal variations, and variations within any one individual, is that pharmacokinetic data gathered in any one study are highly variable. Data gathered from a particular group of persons under a given set of circumstances may not be applicable to another group of persons subjected to a different situation. All this is rather depressing, and has profound implications for the use of any kinetic data.

- Kinetic data listed in appendix-A should not be considered as any more than an approximation of the kinetic parameters of these drugs used in any given individual or population.

- The results of any calculation made using data in appendix-A should therefore not be considered as being any more than an approximation of the expected value.

- If more precision is required from predictions using pharmacokinetic equations, then kinetic data from a group of patients similar to that to which the data are to be applied should be used.

- Chapters 7 to 14 discuss some of the major causes of variation of pharmacokinetic parameters. These discussions provide a basis with which the direction of any change of pharmacokinetic parameters may be predicted.

REFERENCES

1. Woerlee GM: "Common Perioperative Problems and the Anaesthetist", published Kluwer Academic Publishers, 1988, ISBN 0-89838-402-8. pages 508-510.
2. Weigand BD, et al: The use of indocyanine green for the evaluation of hepatic function and blood flow in man. *American Journal of Digestive Diseases*, 1960: 5: 427-436.
3. Ramzan MI, et al: Gallamine disposition in surgical patients with chronic renal failure. *British Journal of Clinical Pharmacology*, 1981: 12: 141-147.
4. Waddell, Bates RG: Intracellular pH. *Physiological Reviews*, 1969: 49: 285-329.
5. Stoekel H, et al: Pharmacokinetics of fentanyl as a possible explanation for delayed recurrence of respiratory depression. *British Journal of Anaesthesia*, 1979: 51: 741-745.
6. Christensen JH, et al: Pharmacokinetics and pharmacodynamics of thiopentone. A comparison between young and elderly patients. *Anaesthesia*, 1982: 37: 398-404.
7. Wagner JG: "Fundamentals of Clinical Pharmacokinetics", published Drug Intelligence Publications Inc., U.S.A., 1979, ISBN 0-914678-20-4.

Chapter 4

Pharmacodynamics

The previous chapter discussed the distribution of an intravenously administered drug within the body. Being able to describe the change of plasma concentration of a drug with time after administration is all very well, but is a rather sterile mathematical pastime to many clinicians. Clinicians are pragmatic people who also want to know if a given dose of a drug will have an effect, and how long that effect is likely to last.

The answers to these questions are provided by pharmacodynamics. Pharmacodynamics is the study of drug effect in relation to drug concentration.

CONCENTRATION-EFFECT RELATIONSHIP

All clinicians recognize that there is a direct relationship between plasma drug concentration and drug effect. There are two aspects to this relationship.

1.   A drug is administered in order to produce an effect. The chance of that effect occurring is directly proportional to the dose or plasma concentration of that drug.

2.   The magnitude of an effect due to a drug is also directly proportional to the plasma concentration or dose of that drug.

CONCENTRATION & PROBABILITY OF EFFECT

Individuals differ from one another. Plasma drug concentration, or dose at which an effect due to any drug occurs differs from one individual to another. Studies show that the minimum plasma concentration at which a drug exerts an effect is distributed around a mean according to the "normal" statistical distribution. However it is usually more convenient to describe the relationship between plasma drug concentration and the probability of an effect due to that drug with a cumulative probability curve. This type of curve is called a cumulative normal probability function, or logistic curve. Figure 4.1 shows a typical example of such a curve, while figure 4.2 shows two such curves derived from clinical investigation.

Figure 4.1: A curve showing the typical relationship between the plasma concentration of a drug and the percentage probability of a given effect due to that drug. The concentration at which 50% of persons develop a given effect is the C_{p50}, and that at which 95% develop the same effect is the C_{p95}. The term γ is a dimensionless parameter. It is the tangent of the angle made by the ascending part of the curve with the x-axis.

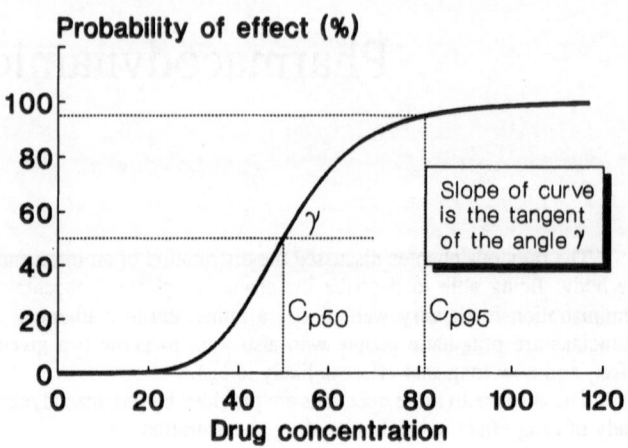

Figure 4.2: Percentage probability of adequate analgesia being present during skin incision and tracheal intubation is directly related to the plasma alfentanil concentration. In the study from which the data for these curves were derived, analgesia was defined as a lack of any significant elevation of blood pressure in response to tracheal intubation or skin incision [16]. This study also showed that the alfentanil concentration required to provide analgesia differed with different stimuli.

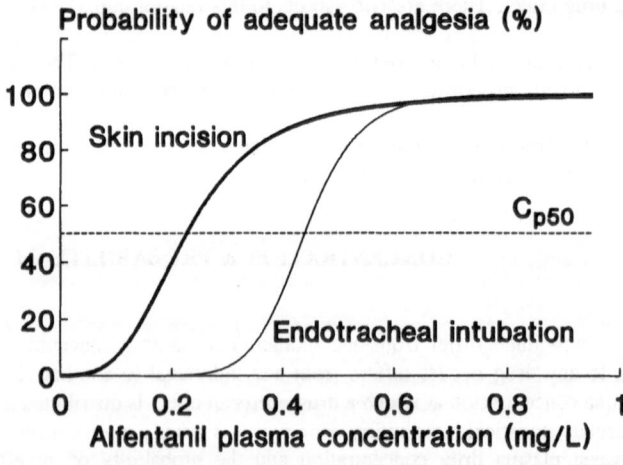

The C_{p50}

Because the initial and terminal parts of the logistic curve are asymptotic, it is very difficult to precisely determine the precise concentration at which an effect begins to manifest, or when it is present in all persons. Accordingly the plasma concentration at which the effect is present in 50% of persons is used. This point is easily determined, and is called the C_{p50}. The C_{p50} is a **median** concentration.

The difference between a "median" and a "mean" value is important in understanding the meaning of the C_{p50}.

- A "mean" value of a variable is an average value. It does not necessarily mean that 50% of a sample have a value of that variable which is less than, and 50% a value greater than the "mean" value of that variable. This is demonstrated in example 4.1.

- A "median" value of a variable is a value at which 50% of persons have a value less than, and 50% of persons have a value greater than the median value of a variable [see example 4.1]. If a variable is normally distributed the "mean" and the "median" are equivalent and can be used interchangeably.

EXAMPLE 4.1:

The difference between "median" and arithmetical "mean" is of fundamental importance. The two concepts should not be confused with each other.

Consider a sample of 6 persons to whom a drug is administered. The minimum plasma drug concentration at which an effect due to that drug occurs is determined for each individual. This minimum plasma concentration is 1, 1.5, 2, 2.5, 5, and 9 mg/L respectively for the six persons. The mean plasma concentration at which the effect occurred is therefore 3.5 mg/L. However, simple inspection shows that the minimum plasma concentration at which 50% of the individuals manifested the effect due to that drug actually lies between 2 and 2.5 mg/L.

In this sample the mean minimum plasma concentration at which the effect due to the drug occurred is quite different to the median minimum plasma concentration at which that effect occurred. If the sample was distributed according to the "normal" distribution they would have been identical.

Slope of curve (γ)

The tangent of the angle that the ascending part of the curve makes with respect to the horizontal at the C_{p50} is the "slope" of the concentration-effect curve. It is usually represented by the greek letter γ. Because slope is the tangent of the angle it is a dimensionless parameter.

Equation of logistic curve

A modified form of the Hill equation is usually used to describe the logistic curve. This is shown below as equation 4.1.

$$\text{Probability of effect} = 1 - \frac{C_{p50}{}^{\gamma}}{C_{p50}{}^{\gamma} + C_p{}^{\gamma}} \qquad (4.1)$$

C_p is the existing plasma concentration of the drug.
C_{p50} is the plasma drug concentration at which the measured effect due to that drug is observed in 50% of persons.
γ is a dimensionless parameter giving the slope of the concentration-effect curve.

The Hill equation in practice, relation of the C_{p50} to the C_{p95}

Equation 4.1, the modified version of the Hill equation can be used to show the relationship between the C_{p50} and the C_{p95}. This relationship has practical clinical uses.

for $\gamma > 2.7$, then $C_{p95} \leq 3 \times C_{p50}$

The value of γ of many drugs used in anesthesia is greater than 2.7. So most anesthetic drugs will exert an effect in 95% of persons when their concentration is about 2-3 times the C_{p50} for that effect. This makes the C_{p50} a clinically useful pharmacodynamic variable [see discussion below on the MEC, and see chapter 6 for examples].

MINIMUM EFFECTIVE CONCENTRATION (MEC)

Most published data relating a minimum plasma drug concentration to an effect are not presented as a C_{p50} or MEDIAN plasma concentration at which that effect occurs. Instead most such data are given as the MEAN minimum plasma drug concentration at which that effect occurs. The distinction is not only statistical, but also in the method of measurement.

- The minimum MEAN plasma concentration at which a drug produces a given effect is measured by determining the minimum plasma concentration at which that effect occurs in each of a number of patients. These data are then pooled to calculate a MEAN concentration.

- The MEDIAN plasma concentration for an effect due to a drug is found by determining the plasma drug concentration at which 50% of persons develop that effect due to that drug.

Despite the essential difference between the MEDIAN plasma concentration and the minimum MEAN plasma concentration at which a given effect due to a drug occurs, these two terms are equivalent when the data on which they are based are normally distributed. Pharmacodynamic data are nearly always normally distributed, and so for all practical purposes these two terms may be considered to be equivalent.

Definition of the MEC

The above discussion means that a clinical pharmacodynamic variable can be defined. This is the Minimum mean Effective plasma Concentration (MEC) at which a given effect due to a drug is observed. It is evident from the discussion above that the MEC is equivalent to the median plasma concentration, or C_{p50} at which an effect due to a drug occurs.

Any one drug may induce a variety of effects. Each of these effects may have a different MEC [see table 4.1].

Table 4.1
MEC of various clinical effects due to some anesthetic induction agents.

Clinical Effect	THIOPENTAL MEC for clinical effect (mg/L)	METHOHEXITAL MEC for clinical effect (mg/L)	ETOMIDATE MEC for clinical effect (mg/L)
Hypnosis	10^{11}	3.4^{13}	0.21^{15}
Loss of eyelid reflex	23^{10}	4.4^{13}	0.46^{15}
Loss of cornea reflex	39^{10}	6.5^{13}	0.65^{15}
Loss of response to pain	40^{10}	?	?
Myocardial depression	70^{12}	10^{14}	15^{12}

Clinical utility of the MEC

The MEC of an effect due to a given drug is not a clinically very useful variable. It is a concentration at which only 50% of persons have developed that effect, while the remaining 50% require a plasma drug concentration which is higher than the MEC if they are to develop that effect. However, because of the equivalence of the C_{p50} and the MEC, a plasma drug concentration which is 2-3 times higher than the MEC will produce that effect in nearly all persons, [see discussion on the relationship between the C_{p50} and the C_{p95}].

EXAMPLE 4.2:

Consider the analgesic drug alfentanil. The C_{p50} = MEC for inhibition of hemodynamic responses to surgical skin incision = 0.23 mg/L, and γ = 3.3 [16]. According to the properties of the C_{p50} or the MEC, a plasma alfentanil concentration which is 3 x C_{p50} = 3 x MEC = 3 x 0.23 mg/L = 0.69 mg/L should be sufficient to block hemodynamic responses to skin incision in more than 95% of patients. This has been confirmed experimentally [16].

CONCENTRATION & MAGNITUDE OF EFFECT

The purpose of this section is to discuss the relationship between drug concentration and magnitude of drug effect.

General properties of any concentration-effect relationship

There are several properties of the relationship between the concentration of a drug and the magnitudes of any effects it exerts which must be explained by any pharmacodynamic model used. These properties are a consequence of the mechanisms of actions of the drugs under consideration. In the case of intravenous anesthetic drugs, all of these drugs act either on a single enzyme or specific receptor sites. The pharmacodynamic consequences of this are listed below.

1. If no drug is present no effect due to that drug will occur.

2. A measurable effect of a drug only will occur after a minimum or threshold drug concentration is present in the target tissues, or a threshold percentage of the receptors or enzyme molecules affected by that drug are blocked or stimulated by that drug. A good example of this are the nondepolarizing muscle relaxants, which must achieve a synaptic concentration sufficient to block at least 70% of the peripheral muscle acetylcholine receptors if they are to cause any measurable skeletal muscle weakness [3,4].

3. For any drug concentration above the minimum or threshold concentration, the magnitude of the drug effect is directly proportional to the dose or concentration of that drug. Drug concentration determines the percentage of available receptors or enzyme molecules that are occupied by drug molecules.

4. All the drug groups listed in table 4.2 have an effect which increases to a maximum with increasing drug concentration. No effect above this maximum effect can be induced by these drugs, not even by administration of huge doses of these drugs. The reason for such a maximum is simple. There are only a finite number of drug receptor sites to be blocked or

stimulated. The same applies to the finite number of molecules of an enzyme which can be stimulated or blocked. Once all these are all stimulated or blocked, there are simply no more receptors or enzyme molecules which can be affected by the drug under consideration. This idea of a maximum effect applies to all the intravenous anesthetic drugs.

Table 4.2.
Mechanisms of action of some drugs used in anesthesia.

Barbiturates	- Increase nerve cell membrane chloride channel conductance.
Benzodiazepines	- Benzodiazepine receptor agonists.
Flumazenil	- Benzodiazepine receptor antagonist.
Opiates	- Opiate receptor agonists.
Opiate antagonists	- Opiate receptor antagonists.
Nondepolarizing relaxants	- Nicotinic acetylcholine receptor antagonists.
Depolarizing relaxants	- Nicotinic acetylcholine receptor agonists.
Anticholinergics	- Muscarinic acetylcholine receptor antagonists.
Anticholinesterases	- Block acetylcholinesterase in both muscarinic and nicotinic acetylcholinergic synapses.

Sigmoid E_{max} model

The concentration-effect relationship of all the intravenous anesthetic drugs may be described using a sigmoid curve. An example of such a curve is shown in figure 4.3, and is described by the Hill equation, [equation 4.2].

$$E = \frac{E_{max} \cdot C^\gamma}{EC_{50}{}^\gamma + C^\gamma} \qquad (4.2)$$

E_{max} is the magnitude of the maximum effect able to be exerted by the drug.
EC_{50} is the concentration of the drug causing an effect whose magnitude is 50% of the maximum possible effect.
C is the drug concentration at any particular moment.
E is the magnitude of the effect due to the drug whose concentration at the time of measuring that effect was equal to C.
γ is a parameter which describes the slope of the curve, and is experimentally determined.

Figure 4.3: This curve shows the concentration-effect relationship which is applicable to all intravenously administered drugs used in anesthesia. Because of the asymptotic nature of the concentration-effect curve at the lower and higher concentration ranges, the EC_{50} is used to describe the **potency**, or effect due to a given concentration of a drug. The **slope**, or tangent of the angle that the curve makes with respect to the x-axis at the EC_{50} point is a measure of the change of drug effect per unit change of drug concentration.

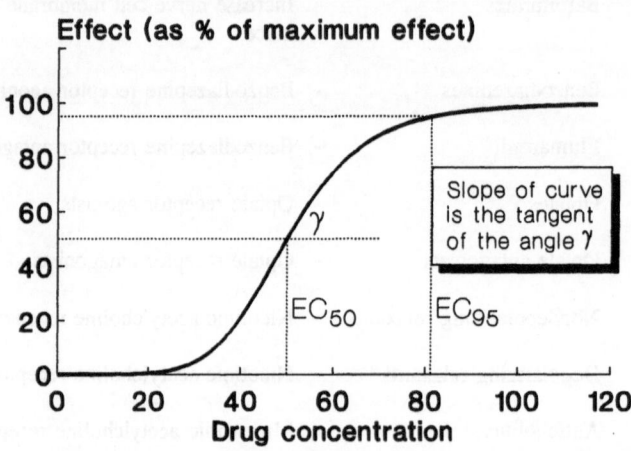

This model explains all the properties required to explain the consequences of the mechanisms of action of intravenous drugs used in anesthesia. There is a maximum drug effect, and a minimum drug concentration must be present before any significant effect occurs. In addition to this, drug effect is directly proportional to the drug concentration. The concentration-effect curves of various non-depolarizing muscle relaxants are shown in figure 4.4 as an example of how this relationship applies to an extensively studied group of drugs.

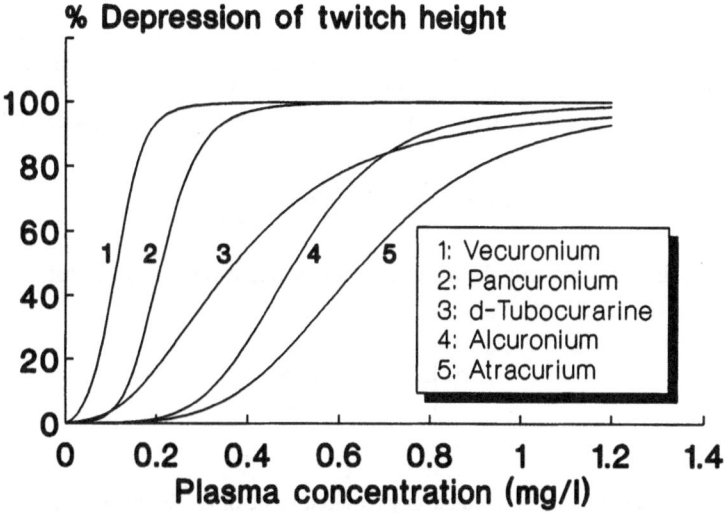

Figure 4.4: Concentration-effect curves of 5 non-depolarizing muscle relaxant drugs [data derived from reference 5].

Table 4.3.

RELAXANT [data from 5]	EC$_{50}$ (mg/L)	γ
Alcuronium	0.5	4.9
Atracurium	0.65	4.2
Gallamine	5.4	4.8
Metocurine	0.29	4
Pancuronium	0.21	5.5
Tubocurarine	0.37	2.6
Vecuronium	0.11	4.9

Use of sigmoid E_{max} equation

EC_{50} and γ are pharmacodynamic variables which can be used to calculate the drug concentration required to produce any magnitude of effect of that drug.

Let $f_{max} = E/E_{max}$, i.e. the fraction of the maximal drug effect, and equation 4.2 becomes;

$$f_{max} = \frac{E}{E_{max}} = \frac{C^\gamma}{EC_{50}^\gamma + C^\gamma} \tag{4.3}$$

Rearrange this equation with the aid of logarithms, and it can be shown that;

$$C = \left[\frac{f_{max}}{1-f_{max}}\right]^{\frac{1}{\gamma}} \times EC_{50} \tag{4.4}$$

Equation 4.4 can be used to calculate any required value of C. Example 4.3 shows one of the uses of equation 4.4.

EXAMPLE 4.3:

Calculate the plasma concentration of pancuronium that only causes 25% of the maximum degree of skeletal muscle paralysis (100%).

- $f_{max} = 0.25$.
- EC_{50} of pancuronium = 0.21 mg/L [table 4.3].
- $\gamma = 5.5$ [table 4.3].
- Substitute these values into equation 4.4 to get C = 0.17 mg/L.

Slope of concentration-effect curve

The slope of the concentration-effect curve is a pharmacodynamic property which is of importance in defining the concentration-effect relationship of a drug [6]. Slopes of drug concentration-effect curves differ. Some drugs have a **low-slope** curve and others a **high-slope** curve. The slope of the concentration-effect curve of a drug has clinical consequences.

- The effect of any given change of concentration of a high-slope drug is greater than that were the same drug to have a low-slope concentration-effect curve.

- Duration of clinical effect of a drug with a given EC_{50}, $t_{1/2\alpha}$ and $t_{1/2\beta}$ is inversely related to the slope of the concentration-effect curve of that drug. So if a given drug has a low-slope concentration-effect curve it will produce a longer lasting clinical effect than were that same drug to have a high-slope concentration-effect curve, [see figures 4.5 and 4.6]. There are drugs used in clinical practice which have similar elimination and distribution half lives, but whose concentration-effect curves have very different slopes. Two such drugs are pancuronium and d-tubocurarine, and the consequence of their having differing concentration-effect curve slopes is shown in example 4.4 and figure 4.6.

Figure 4.5: This figure shows the consequences of differing slopes of concentration-effect curves for a drug. As it is the same drug for both curves, EC_{50}, $t_{1/2\alpha}$ and $t_{1/2\beta}$ are the same for both curves. C_1 and C_2 show a concentration range in which the drug concentration may be considered to either halve or double. It is apparent that if the drug has a **high-slope curve** that the effect of the drug changes from nothing to maximum in the concentration range C_1 to C_2. But if the same drug had a **low-slope curve** the effect would not be maximum at C_2, and would still be significant at C_1.

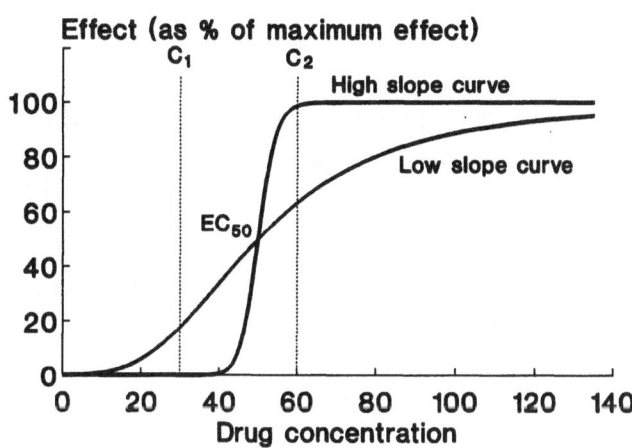

EXAMPLE 4.4:

Pancuronium is a drug with a high-slope concentration-effect curve, while d-tubocurarine has a low-slope concentration-effect curve.

Consider a person who was administered a single intravenous dose of d-tubocurarine on one day and pancuronium on another day. The doses were such that at the end of their respective distribution phases the plasma concentration of pancuronium was 0.36 mg/L, and that of d-tubocurarine was 1.18 mg/L. Concentrations of both drugs were sufficient to reduce muscle contraction strength to only 5% of normal, [see reference 5, or use equation 4.4 and table 4.3]. These initial plasma concentrations are shown in figure 4.6 as T_1 for d-tubocurarine and P_1 for pancuronium. Because the distribution phases of both drugs were complete, the only way plasma and effect compartment drug concentrations could decrease was by drug elimination.

The elimination half lives of pancuronium and d-tubocurarine are about the same, being 114 and 119 minutes respectively. After one elimination half life, the drug concentrations of both pancuronium and d-tubocurarine had halved to 0.18 mg/L and 0.59 mg/L respectively. These concentrations meant that pancuronium exerted an effect that was 30% of maximum, and d-tubocurarine exerted an effect which was 77% of maximum, [use equation 4.4 and table 4.3 to calculate this]. Quite a difference!

This difference between these two kinetically similar drugs is purely due to their different concentration-effect curve slopes. So while d-tubocurarine has essentially the same kinetic properties as pancuronium, it has a longer duration of action than an equivalent dose of pancuronium.

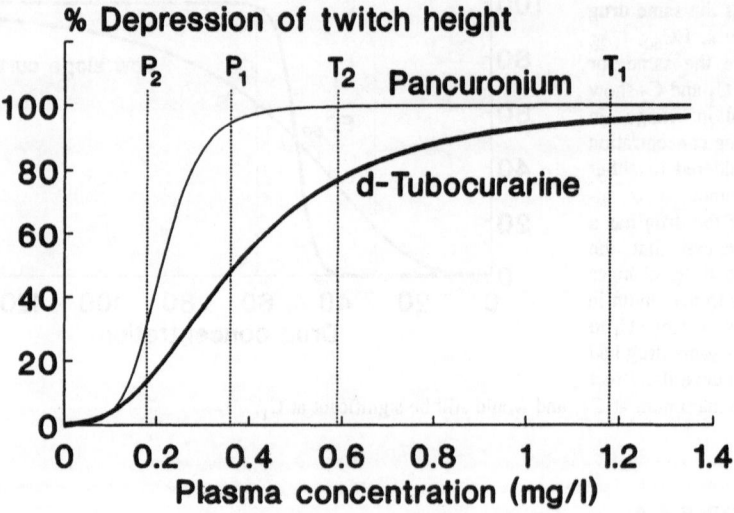

Figure 4.6: Pancuronium is a "high-slope" drug while d-tubocurarine is a "low-slope" drug. Both drugs have approximately the same $t_{1/2\beta}$. In this example, a single intravenous dose of each of these drugs was administered at different times to the same person. The doses were sufficient so that after completion of the distribution phase, both the plasma and effect compartment concentrations were high enough to reduce muscle strength to only 5% of normal. The consequences of the different concentration-effect curve slopes of these drugs is discussed in example 4.4. .

Concentration-effect curve slope, half lives and the ideal anesthetic drug

Example 4.4, and figures 4.5 and 4.6 show that the slope of the concentration-effect curve should never be considered separately from the $t_{1/2\beta}$ or the $t_{1/2\alpha}$. The speed with which the effect of a drug is terminated is a function of both slope and the rate of change of effect compartment drug concentration [6].

The ideal anesthetic drug is one with a high-slope concentration-effect curve. The advantage of this is that the effect of the drug is terminated very rapidly once the plasma drug concentration falls below a given critical concentration. This means that the effect of the drug can be maintained at a maximal level until either redistribution or elimination reduces the drug concentration below this critical level [7]. An example of this is shown in figure 4.5. The critical concentration in figure 4.5 is C_2. Such a drug will act as if it only produces a maximal or no effect, a very useful property for hypnotic, opiate or muscle relaxant drugs.

Slope and drug sensitivity

"Sensitivity" is a term which is commonly used to describe the reaction of an individual to a particular drug. A person is **sensitive** to a particular drug when the clinical response to a given dose, or change of concentration of that drug is greater than normal. Such a phenomenon has two explanations.

- The slope of a concentration-effect curve for any particular drug varies from one individual to another. Some persons have a steeper curve than others. Those individuals with a concentration-response curve which is steep relative to that of other persons for the same drug, will manifest a greater clinical effect in response to any given dose of that drug.

- Because of the sigmoid shape of the concentration-effect relationship, an effect resulting from any dose of a drug depends very much on the existing drug concentration and the drug dose. Consider the situation of a drug with a high-slope concentration effect curve. If the drug concentration is such that 50% of the maximum possible effect is present, then the person will manifest a large response to any small incremental dose of that drug. The person is "sensitive" to that drug at that concentration because the curve is steepest at this point. But if the existing concentration of that drug was so low that the drug effect was nearly non-existent, or so high that the effect was nearly maximum, then the same small incremental drug dose will have very little effect. A person is not very sensitive to the effects of that drug in these concentration ranges because the concentration-effect curve slope is low in these ranges. Figure 4.3 shows these points well.

Hyperbolic E_{max} model

If $g = 1$ in the sigmoid E_{max} model equation, then the resulting equation is that of a **hyperbola** whose origin is at concentration $= 0$ [equation 4.5]

$$E = \frac{E_{max} \cdot C}{EC_{50} + C} \tag{4.5}$$

Such a hyperbolic equation may be used to describe the concentration-effect curves of drugs in a concentration range where the drug concentration is greater than the minimum required for any effect. In other words, this model can be used to describe a part of a concentration-effect curve which otherwise is described fully by a sigmoid E_{max} model. An example of a drug whose pharmacodynamics may be described with such an equation is theophylline in the plasma concentration range 4-22 mg/L [8].

Linear model

The middle part of the sigmoid E_{max} curve is approximately linear. In this concentration range the concentration-effect relationship of a drug may be approximated with a simple linear equation.

$$E = a + b.C \tag{4.6}$$

a and b are experimentally derived constants.
E and C have their usual meanings.

EXAMPLE 4.5:

An example of the practical application of a linear model is given by equation 4.7. Equation 4.7 is an experimentally derived linear equation describing the effect of d-tubocurarine on skeletal muscle contraction strength in the plasma concentration range 0.2-0.7 mg/L [9]. This is a concentration range in which the sigmoid curve is approximately linear [see figure 4.6].

$$\text{Contraction Strength (\% control)} = 146 - 212.C_{dtc} \tag{4.7}$$

C_{dtc} is the plasma d-tubocurarine concentration in mg/L.

Fixed effect relationship

In most clinical situations drugs are administered in doses which are clinically effective. Any lesser effect is classified as ineffective. Such situations occur throughout clinical medicine and within anesthetic practice too, e.g. the use of antibiotics, muscle relaxants, opiates, antiarrhythmic drugs, etc. This is called a "fixed effect" relationship. Such a relationship is also described by a sigmoid E_{max} curve with an extremely high slope, i.e. where the angle that the curve makes with the x-axis at the EC_{50} is approximately 90°.

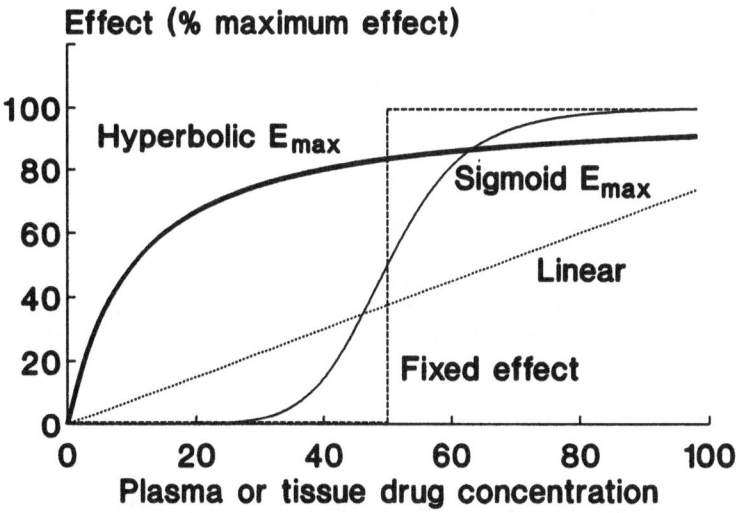

Figure 4.7: This figure shows the general forms of the concentration-effect curves of the hyperbolic E_{max}, sigmoid E_{max}, linear and fixed effect pharmacodynamic models.

PHARMACOKINETIC - DYNAMIC MODELLING

Anesthetic drugs do not exert their effects by acting on blood. Instead they act on cells which are situated outside blood vessels. So the relationship between plasma drug concentration and effect which has been discussed in the previous pages is only valid for plasma drug concentrations which have been maintained at a constant level long enough for a blood-tissue drug concentration equilibrium to have occurred. Such a situation never occurs when blood drug concentrations are continuously changing. A pharmacokinetic-dynamic model is necessary to account for drug effects for the situation of continuously changing blood drug concentrations.

Entry of drug into effector organs

Rate of entry of drugs into perivascular tissues is determined by several factors [see chapter 2].

- The rate with which a drug diffuses into extravascular tissues is inversely proportional to the molecular weight of the drug.

- Fat-soluble drugs diffuse more rapidly out of capillaries than fat-insoluble drugs.

- Blood concentration of the drug determines the plasma-tissue concentration gradient.

- The rate with which drugs diffuse or flow into extravascular tissues is directly proportional to the plasma-tissue concentration gradient.

All these factors mean that no drug is active in the instant it arrives at the organs where it is active. A drug must first leave the blood vessels and arrive at the cells where it is active. It must also be present in, or around these cells at a concentration sufficient to exert an effect.

Tissue concentration - effect relationship

Magnitude of drug effect is directly proportional to drug concentration in the tissues where the drug is active. The time required for a drug to exert an effect whose magnitude is related to a given tissue drug concentration is a function of the mechanism of action of that drug. Intravenously administered drugs used in anesthetic practice usually act by stimulating or blocking specific receptors or enzymes. Drug-receptor, and drug-enzyme interactions require only fractions of a second, and so may be considered to be instantaneous.

Effect compartment

All the factors causing a delay of drug effect after achieving a given blood drug concentration can be modelled quite well by postulating a "biophase" [1] or "effect" [2] compartment where the drug exerts its effect. This effect compartment is coupled to other pharmacokinetic compartments [see figure 4.8]. A multicompartment pharmacokinetic model coupled to an effect compartment has two very practical advantages.

- Changes of drug concentration in the effect compartment can be modelled using a familiar multicompartment model.

- The actual volume of the effect compartment is difficult to measure. However the volume of the effect compartment is irrelevant if only differential equations are used to calculate drug concentrations.

Temporal relation between blood drug concentration and effect

An effect compartment model also explains the temporal relation between a given plasma drug concentration and drug effect related to that concentration.

- It takes time for a given quantity of any drug to diffuse from the blood into the effect compartment, and vice versa. This means that there us always a time difference between achieving a given plasma drug concentration and the drug effect related to that drug concentration.

- Once a drug is inside the effect compartment, the assumption is made that the drug effect related to a given concentration of a drug may be considered to occur instantaneously. This means that the delay of a drug effect related to a given plasma drug concentration of a drug is due to the time required for the drug to achieve the same concentration in the effect compartment.

3-Compartment kinetic-dynamic model

Figure 4.8: A 2-compartment pharmacokinetic model is shown coupled to an **effect compartment**. The effect compartment exchanges drug with compartment-1 and behaves otherwise in the same way as a pharmacokinetic compartment. Such a model can be modelled using a 3-compartment kinetic model.

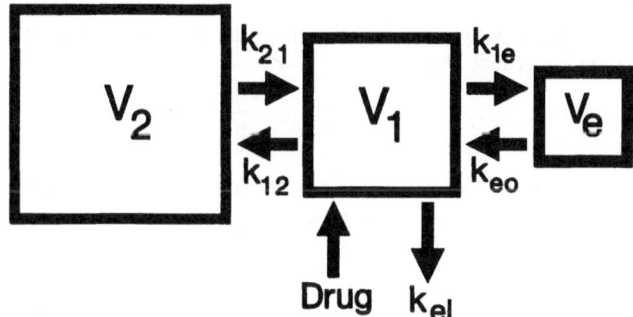

An effect compartment model

Figure 4.8 shows an effect compartment coupled to a standard 2-compartment pharmacokinetic model. The effect compartment behaves in exactly the same way as any pharmacokinetic compartment, and the mathematical treatment is also identical. This chapter will concentrate on this particular 3-compartment model as it adequately describes the behavior of nearly all anesthetic drugs.

Despite the third effect compartment, the kinetics of a drug are still able to be well described by a 2-compartment model, as several assumptions are made about the properties of this compartment [2].

- The volume of the effect compartment is insignificantly small in comparison with the volumes of the other two compartments. So it also contains a negligibly small proportion of the total amount of drug present in the body at any one time. This is demonstrated by the fact that drug kinetics are able to be described by a 2-, instead of a 3-compartment model.

- The rate of transfer of drug (k_{1e}) to the effect compartment from the central compartment is small in relation to all other kinetic rate constants.

- Because k_{1e} is negligibly small, the rate of change of drug concentration in the effect compartment is primarily determined by the rate constant for drug elimination from the effect compartment, k_{eo}.

The relationship describing the rate of change of drug concentration in the effect compartment can be derived using the principles discussed in chapter 1. This given by equation 4.8.

$$\frac{dC_e}{dt} = C_1.k_{1e} - C_e.k_{eo} \qquad (4.8)$$

As k_{1e} is very small in relation to the other rate constants in the 2-compartment model, equation 4.1 reduces to;

$$\frac{dC_e}{dt} = -C_e.k_{eo} \qquad (4.9)$$

However rate of change of concentration only affects the **DIFFERENCE** in concentration between C_1 and C_e, and is not related to C_e alone. So equation 4.9 must be rewritten as equation 4.10.

$$\frac{dC_e}{dt} = - (C_e - C_1)k_{eo} = k_{eo}(C_1 - C_e) \qquad (4.10)$$

Equation 4.10 is very useful for calculating effect compartment concentrations when this is rapidly changing. It is used extensively for this purpose in the next chapters. The exact solutions of equation 4.10 giving the effect compartment drug concentration for the two situations of drug diffusing into and out of this compartment are;

Drug diffusing **INTO** effect compartment

$$C_e = C_{eo} + (C - C_{eo})(1 - e^{-keo.t}) \qquad (4.11)$$

Drug diffusing **OUT OF** effect compartment

$$C_e = C + (C_{eo} - C)e^{-keo.t} \qquad (4.12)$$

t is time.
C is the plasma drug concentration which is assumed to be constant and unchanging.

C_{eo} is the effect compartment concentration at time $= 0$.
C_e is the effect compartment drug concentration after a given time has elapsed.

Half life of plasma-effect compartment drug exchange

As k_{eo} is a rate constant of an exponential equation to the base "e" it may also be expressed as a half life [see chapter 1, equation 1.10]. This half life is termed the $t_{1/2}k_{eo}$ and is defined by equation 4.13.

$$t_{1/2}k_{eo} = \frac{0.693}{k_{eo}} \qquad (4.13)$$

Appendix A lists known values of $t_{1/2}k_{eo}$ for various anesthetic drugs. Inspection of these values for $t_{1/2}k_{eo}$ reveals that they are of the same order of magnitude as the half lives of plasma-tissue concentration equilibrium known for other substances with similar molecular weights [see chapter 2].

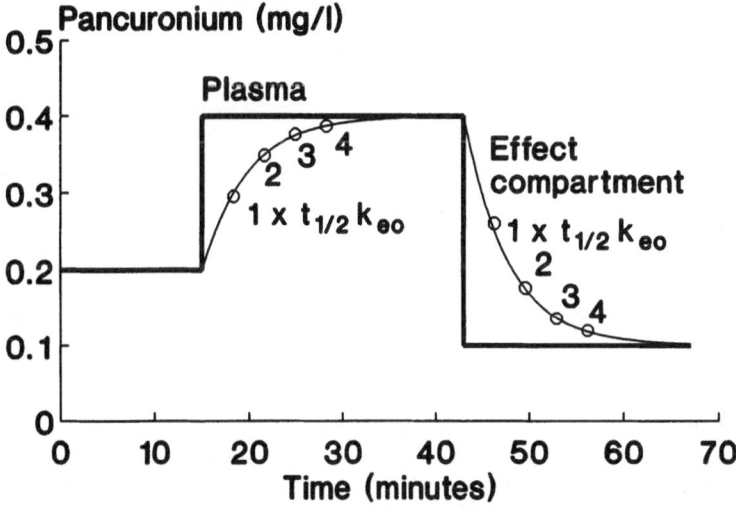

Figure 4.9: In the first 15 minutes of this figure, plasma- and effect compartment pancuronium concentrations are equal. Plasma pancuronium concentration is then instantaneously increased to a new constant level, and later instantaneously decreased to another new constant level. In both situations it takes time before the effect compartment concentration equals the plasma concentration because the drug must diffuse into, or out of the effect compartment. This figure also shows that regardless of the magnitude of change of plasma drug concentration, it always takes about 4 times the $t_{1/2}k_{eo}$ before plasma- and effect compartment drug concentrations equalize.

Speed of plasma-effect compartment drug concentration equilibrium

The rate at which the effect compartment drug concentration approaches an equilibrium with that in blood or plasma is determined by the $t_{1/2}k_{eo}$. Because the $t_{1/2}k_{eo}$ is a half life, this means that for the situation of a constant blood drug concentration, that the achievement of an equilibrium between plasma and the effect compartment is nearly complete in a time equivalent to 4 times the $t_{1/2}k_{eo}$ for any particular drug [see chapter 1, table 1.1 in section on "Natural logarithms and half life", and figure 4.9].

The speed with which a drug in the plasma diffuses into the effect compartment has clinical consequences. It is this which determines the speed of onset of drug effect. This is illustrated by examples 4.6 and 4.7 [see also figures 4.10 and 4.11].

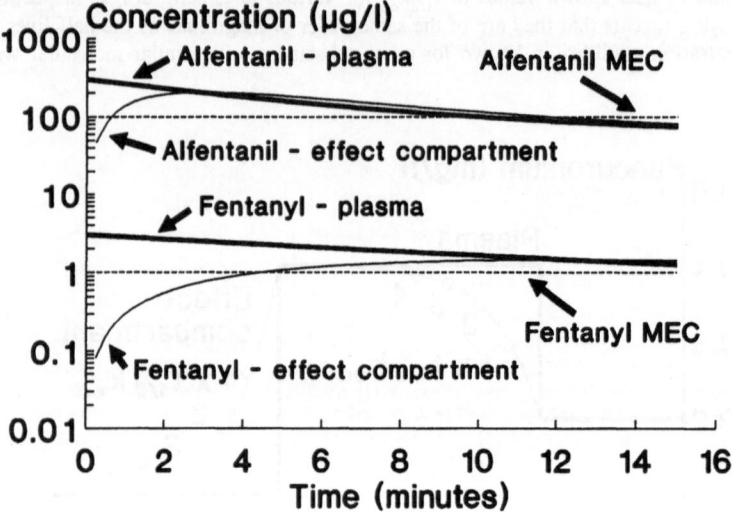

Figure 4.10: Plasma and effect compartment concentration time curves are shown for single intravenous doses of fentanyl 2.31 μg/kg (= 0.16 mg for an adult), and alfentanil 51.02 μg/kg (= 3.5 mg for an adult). The doses of both opiates are such that their initial plasma concentrations are three times their MEC for postoperative analgesia. Alfentanil has a shorter $t_{1/2}k_{eo}$ than does fentanyl. So an equivalent, or equipotent dose of alfentanil acts sooner than fentanyl.

EXAMPLE 4.6:

Consider the administration of single intravenous doses of fentanyl 2.31 μg/kg (= 0.16 mg for an adult), and of alfentanil 51.02 μg/kg (= 3.5 mg in an adult). The dose of each drug is just sufficient to provide an initial plasma concentration of the opiate which is three times greater than the MEC for postoperative analgesia of each opiate. This can be calculated using equations 3.20, 3.36 or 3.38 [see appendix-A for data].

Fentanyl

- MEC of fentanyl for postoperative analgesia = 1 μg/L.
- Dose = 2.31 μg/kg.
- A = dose x A_x = 2.31 x 1.09 = 2.52 μg/l.
- B = dose x B_x = 2.31 x 0.21 = 0.48 μg/l.
- The initial plasma fentanyl concentration = C = A + B = 2.52 + 0.48 = 3 μg/l. This is three times the MEC of fentanyl for postoperative analgesia.

Alfentanil

- MEC of alfentanil for postoperative analgesia = 100 μg/l.
- Dose = 51.02 μg/kg.
- A = dose x A_x = 51.02 x 4.24 = 216.32 μg/l.
- B = dose x B_x = 51.02 x 1.64 = 83.67 μg/l.
- The initial plasma alfentanil concentration = C = A + B = 216.32 + 83.67 = 300 μg/l. This is three times the MEC of alfentanil for postoperative analgesia.

$t_{1/2}k_{eo}$ *and Consequences*

- Fentanyl $t_{1/2}k_{eo}$ = 6.4 minutes.
- Alfentanil $t_{1/2}k_{eo}$ = 1.1 minutes.

As the initial plasma concentrations of both drugs relative to their minimum effective concentrations are identical, it is the difference between the $t_{1/2}k_{eo}$ of both drugs which determines the relative speed of onset of analgesia of each drug. Alfentanil has a shorter $t_{1/2}k_{eo}$ than fentanyl, which means that it can diffuse more rapidly into the effect compartment, and so the analgesic effect of alfentanil manifests sooner than that of a comparable dose of fentanyl.

Opiates are administered by the anesthetist during surgical procedures to blunt autonomic responses such as hypertension and tachycardia which occur in response to the pain of surgery. Fentanyl and alfentanil are popular opiates for this purpose. The longer $t_{1/2}k_{eo}$ of fentanyl means that it is not the most effective opiate to administer in response to an acute requirement for analgesia, as the speed of onset of analgesia is slower than for a comparable dose of alfentanil.

The situation discussed in example 4.6 is also applicable to other drugs, and not only opiates.

Dose and speed of onset of drug effect

Speed of onset of drug affect is directly proportional to drug dose. This is because the rate of diffusion of a drug into the effect compartment is directly proportional to the plasma-to-effect compartment concentration difference, which in turn is directly proportional to the drug dose.

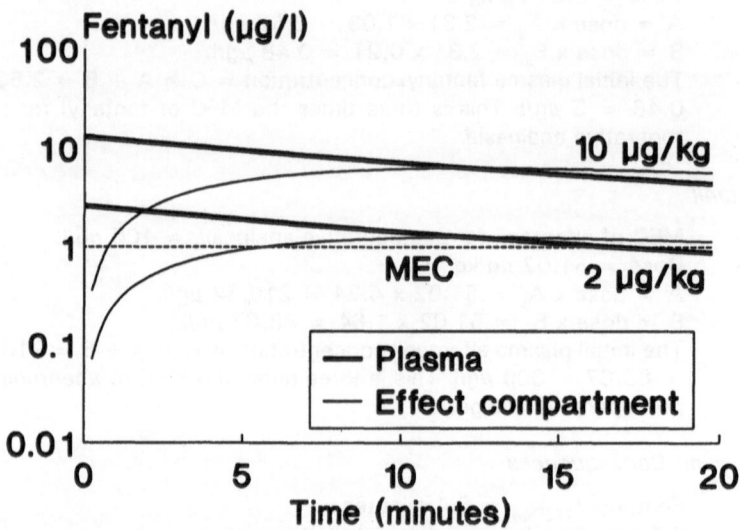

Figure 4.11: Plasma and effect compartment concentration-time curves are shown for two doses of fentanyl, one of 2 $\mu g/kg$ (=0.15 mg for an adult), and another of 10 $\mu g/kg$ (=0.7 mg for an adult). This figure also shows the relationship of the curves to MEC of fentanyl for postoperative analgesia. These curves show that the higher the dose, the more rapidly the effect compartment concentration rises to the desired level.

EXAMPLE 4.7:

Consider two single intravenous doses of fentanyl. One dose of 2 $\mu g/kg$, and one of 10 $\mu g/kg$. The changes of plasma and effect compartment fentanyl concentrations with time after these doses has been simulated in figure 4.11 using equations 3.40 and 4.10. These curves show what is known by all practical clinicians. Time to onset of drug effect for any drug is shorter with higher drug doses, and vice versa.

TIME TO ONSET OF DRUG ACTION

A drug only begins to cause an effect whose magnitude is related to the plasma concentration of that drug when the effect compartment drug concentration is equal to the plasma concentration of that drug. It is known that plasma and effect compartment drug concentrations are nearly equal after the plasma drug concentration has been constant for at least 4 times the $t_{1/2}k_{eo}$. However this is a situation which is seldom achieved during anesthesia, especially when drugs are administered intermittently. So the following considerations must always be kept in mind.

- If the plasma drug concentration is increasing, the effect compartment drug concentration is lower than that in the plasma. So a given drug effect will occur at a plasma drug concentration which is higher than that expected from the MEC for that effect.

- If the plasma drug concentration is decreasing the situation is reversed. Now the effect compartment drug concentration is higher than that in the plasma. A given drug effect will occur at a plasma drug concentration which is lower than that expected from the MEC for that effect.

These relationships are illustrated in figures 4.9 and 4.13. Known MEC values of drugs commonly used in anesthesia are listed in tables 4.3, 5.1, and appendix-A.

The time taken for the drug effect to develop after the plasma drug concentration has been suddenly elevated to "C" can be derived for the special case where the initial plasma and effect compartment drug concentrations are zero. Let $C_{eo} = 0$, and substitute MEC for C_e in equation 4.11 to get equation 4.14:

$$MEC = C \times (1 - e^{-keo.t}) \qquad (4.14)$$

Rearrange equation 4.14 and use the properties of logarithms to get equation 4.15.

$$t_e = -\frac{\ln(1 - MEC/C)}{k_{eo}} = -\frac{t_{1/2}k_{eo}.\ln(1 - MEC/C)}{0.693} \qquad (4.15)$$

t_e is the time required for drug effect to occur if the plasma drug concentration is suddenly elevated to "C".

Equation 4.15 is rather complicated. Computation may be simplified by letting part of the equation be a constant and using a table. Part of equation 4.15 may therefore be defined as a constant "k_{mec}";

$$k_{mec} = \frac{\ln(1 - MEC/C)}{0.693} \qquad (4.16)$$

and so;

$$t_e = t_{1/2}k_{eo} \times k_{mec} \tag{4.17}$$

Values for k_{mec} have been set out in table 4.4.

Table 4.4.

$\dfrac{MEC}{C}$	k_{mec}
0.25	0.42
0.5	1.0
0.75	2.0
1.0	∞

Unfortunately equation 4.17 describes a rather uncommon situation in clinical anesthesia. It assumes a constant plasma or blood drug concentration which has been elevated suddenly to a new constant level. Such a change of drug concentration only occurs during a BET infusion which will be discussed in chapter 6. This is a situation which is almost never encountered in clinical medicine, as the plasma concentration of a newly administered drug is continually changing due to the processes of elimination and distribution. Actual calculation of effect compartment drug concentrations when plasma drug concentrations are changing is a complicated process and will not be engaged in here. However despite the limitations of equation 4.16 it still does provide some insights into the speed of onset of drug effect after a given plasma concentration is achieved. This is illustrated by example 4.8.

EXAMPLE 4.8:

Consider a situation where the plasma concentration of pancuronium is instantly changed from nothing to 0.48 mg/L, and subsequently maintained at that level. How long will it take for the effect compartment concentration to be equal to the MEC of pancuronium? Use the data in appendix-A.

- MEC of pancuronium = the EC_{80} = 0.27 mg/L [see appendix-A for discussion of EC_{80}].
- $t_{1/2}k_{eo}$ of pancuronium = 3.3 minutes.

- Plasma concentration of pancuronium = 0.48 mg/L.
- MEC/C = 0.27/0.48 = 0.56.
- This means that the k_{mec} = 1.3 [equation 4.16].
- Accordingly $t_e = k_{mec} \times t_{1/2}k_{eo}$ = 1.3 x 3.3 = 4.3 minutes. This is the time taken for the effect compartment concentration to equal the MEC. Figure 4.12 shows the change in effect compartment and plasma drug concentrations resulting from such a drug administration scheme.

In actual fact, this method of drug administration corresponds to a BET infusion method, which is at present rather uncommon in routine clinical practice. Pancuronium is usually administered as intermittent intravenous doses. Figure 4.13 shows the rather more complicated changes in plasma and effect compartment concentrations resulting from a single intravenous 4 mg dose of pancuronium, and this brings us to the next discussion point.

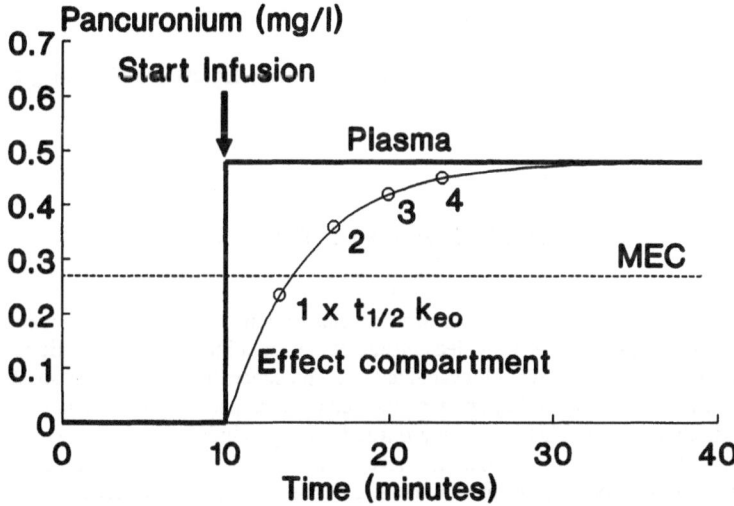

Figure 4.12: The plasma and effect compartment concentration changes with time are shown for the situation where plasma pancuronium concentration is suddenly elevated to, and maintained at 0.48 mg/L. It should be noted that it takes somewhat more than 4 times the $t_{1/2}k_{eo}$ before the effect compartment concentration equals that in the plasma.

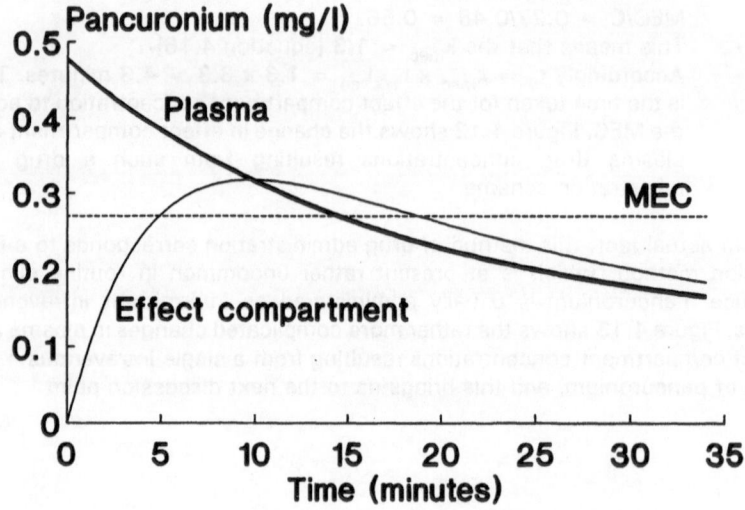

Figure 4.13: Effect compartment and plasma pancuronium concentrations resulting from a single intravenous dose of 4 mg pancuronium.

TIME-EFFECT RELATIONSHIP

The discussion up till this point has been confined mainly to the effects of a constant drug concentration. Now while this has provided considerable insight into kinetic-dynamic relationships, it is not really relevant to the usual clinical situation. The concentrations of most anesthetic drugs are seldom constant except when they are administered by intravenous infusion, and even then, they are not necessarily constant. This is even more true for drugs administered as intravenous boluses, after which plasma drug concentrations are never constant. Plasma drug concentrations change continually due to the processes of distribution and elimination, as well as repeat doses.

The effect of a drug changes due to variations in tissue drug concentration resulting from changing plasma drug concentration. Pharmacodynamic and kinetic equations may be used to calculate the change of drug effect with time after any drug administration method. Predictions made in this way are clinically very relevant, and correspond well with clinical reports on drug effects. This correspondence with clinical effect is actually not surprising. After all, the kinetic and dynamic parameters used in the equations were derived from clinical studies.

An example of the equations, and method required are provided by the equations used for modelling the effects of drugs administered as an intravenous bolus;

$$C = \text{Dose}(A_x.e^{-\alpha t} + B_x.e^{-\beta t}) \tag{3.40}$$

$$\frac{dC_e}{dt} = k_{eo}(C-C_e) \tag{4.10}$$

$$E(\%) = \frac{100 \times E_{max} \times C_e^{\gamma}}{EC_{50}^{\gamma} + C_e^{\gamma}} \tag{4.2}$$

The procedure used is as follows. Use a computer spreadsheet program. In one column, calculate plasma drug concentration (C) with equation 3.40 for every 0.1 minute after drug administration. Euler's method is then used to calculate the effect compartment drug concentration C_e in an adjacent column. This effect compartment drug concentration is then used to calculate the magnitude of the drug effect in the next adjacent column for any given time after a drug dose. The time-effect curves for different doses of popular muscle relaxants have been calculated using this method and are shown in figure 4.14.

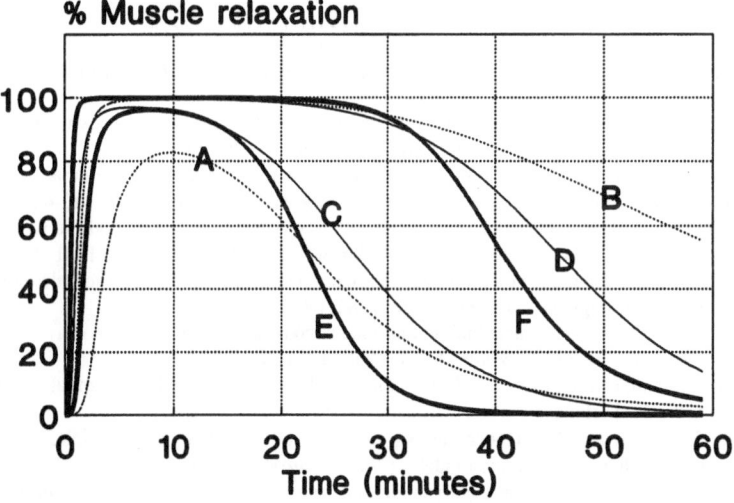

Figure 4.14: This figure shows the muscle relaxant effects of various commonly used dosages of some non-depolarizing relaxants related to time. Curves **A** and **B** are for pancuronium, 0.05 and 0.1 mg/kg respectively. Curves **C** and **D** are for atracurium, 0.25 and 0.5 mg/kg respectively. Curves **E** and **F** are for vecuronium, 0.05 and 0.1 mg/kg respectively. Such curves are typical examples of what is possible with pharmacodynamic modelling.

The procedure outlined above is interesting, but unfortunately cannot be performed without the aid of a computer. As such it is not really a useful tool for use in current clinical anesthetic practice. At this time, the main use for such a calculation procedure is in devising new drug administration schemes for drugs whose kinetic and dynamic properties are known, and for teaching purposes to show how the effect of a drug changes with time after administration.

This may change soon. Real-time computer registration of drug administration is a definite possibility in the near future. Prototype systems are already being tested. In such situations, a kinetic-dynamic modelling program may be concurrently used as part of an expert system to allow more precise anesthetic drug administration.

A FINAL NOTE

This concludes the discussion of drug dynamics. Readers should note that this chapter has not dealt with the subject of drug interactions. This is unfortunate, however the reason for this omission is simple. Drug-drug interactions is a large and complex subject in its' own right, and is out of place in a chapter which strives only to impart a basic knowledge of pharmacodynamic theory.

REFERENCES

1.   Hull CJ, et al: A pharmacodynamic model for pancuronium. *British Journal of Anaesthesia*, 1978: 50: 1113-1123.
2.   Sheiner LB, et al: Simultaneous modelling of pharmacokinetics and pharmacodynamics: Application to d-tubocurarine. *Clinical Pharmacology & Therapeutics*, 1979: 25: 358-371.
3.   Waud BE, Waud DR: The relation between the response to "train-of-four" stimulation and receptor occlusion during competitive neuromuscular block. *Anesthesiology*, 1972: 37: 413-416.
4.   Yodlowski EH, Mortimer JT: The relationship between receptor occlusion and the frequency sweep electromyogram during competitive neuromuscular blockade. *Anesthesiology*, 1981: 54: 23-28.
5.   Shanks CA: Pharmacokinetics of the nondepolarizing neuromuscular applied to calculation of bolus and infusion dosage regimes. *Anesthesiology*, 1986: 64: 72-86.
6.   Hennis PJ, Stanski DR: Pharmacokinetic and pharmacodynamic factors that govern the clinical use of muscle relaxants. *Seminars in Anesthesia*, 1985: 4: 21-30.
7.   Personal communication from Professor Dr P.J. Hennis, University Hospital of Groningen, Groningen, the Netherlands.
8.   Holford NHG, Sheiner LB: Understanding the dose effect relationship: Clinical application of pharmacokinetic-pharmacodynamic models. *Clinical Pharmacokinetics*, 1981: 6: 429-453.
9.   Wingard LB, Cook DR: Pharmacodynamics of tubocurarine in humans. *British Journal of Anaesthesia*, 1976: 48: 839-845.
10.   Becker KE: Plasma levels of thiopental necessary for anesthesia. *Anesthesiology*, 1978: 49: 192-196.
11.   Hudson RJ, et al: A model for studying depth of anesthesia and acute tolerance to thiopental. *Anesthesiology*, 1983: 59: 301-308.
12.   Kissin I, et al: Inotropic and anesthetic potencies of etomidate and thiopental in dogs. *Anesthesia and Analgesia*, 1983: 62: 961-965.

13. Lauven PM, et al: Venous threshold concentrations of methohexitone. *Anesthesiology*, 1985: 63: A368.
14. Todd MM, et al: The hemodynamic consequences of high-dose methohexital anesthesia in humans. *Anesthesiology*, 1984: 61: 495-501.
15. Schüttler J, et al: Infusion strategies to investigate the pharmacokinetics and pharmacodynamics of hypnotic drugs: etomidate as an example. *European Journal of Anesthesiology*, 1985: 2: 133-142.
16. Lemmens HJM, et al: Age has no effect on the pharmacodynamics of alfentanil. *Anesthesia and Analgesia*, 1988: 67: 956-960.

Chapter 5

Practical I.V. Bolus Kinetics & Dynamics

The previous four chapters have discussed the basic principles of drug kinetics and dynamics. These principles will be applied in this chapter to explain the known clinical properties of anesthetic drugs administered as intermittent intravenous doses. A drug administered as a single rapid intravenous dose is called a **bolus** intravenous dose.

The kinetic model used in this chapter is the 2-compartment model to which a third effect compartment is added [see chapters 3 and 4].

CALCULATION OF DRUG CONCENTRATIONS

Change of plasma drug concentration with time after bolus intravenous injection may be divided into three phases, the pre-recirculation-, distribution- and elimination phases.

Pre-recirculation phase

The pre-recirculation phase starts immediately after intravenous injection of a drug and lasts until recirculation of blood from the upper body occurs after 20-30 seconds. It is during the pre-recirculation phase that blood drug concentrations are at their highest levels. So despite the brevity of this phase it is of considerable pharmacological importance. Many anesthetic drugs exert a clinically evident, **but not necessarily maximal effect** in this time. Examples of this are induction of hypnosis, cardiovascular and respiratory depression due to thiopental or other anesthetic induction agents. The magnitudes of these effects are directly related to the magnitude of the peak plasma drug concentrations achieved.

Unfortunately it is impossible to derive a simple equation to calculate the peak pre-recirculation phase drug concentrations. Such a simple formula is unlikely to be possible because of all the factors influencing recirculation drug concentrations [see chapter 2 for a more complete discussion]. All that will be done in this chapter is to cite known pre-recirculation phase drug concentrations where appropriate.

Distribution phase

The distribution phase of a drug may for practical purposes be defined as beginning immediately after intravenous administration of that drug. Plasma drug concentration falls rapidly during the distribution phase. This rapid fall of drug concentration is mainly due to drug distribution from the central compartment volume to the whole of the distribution volume of that drug.

Duration of distribution phase

Drug distribution is 93.75% complete after a time $= 4 \times t_{1/2\alpha}$. This can be considered to be the duration of the distribution phase.

Initial drug concentration at time $= 0$

Initial plasma drug concentration at time $= 0$ after bolus injection of a drug is given by equation 3.20.

$$C_0 = A + B \tag{3.20}$$

Drug concentration at time > 0

Distribution begins the moment after a drug is administered. Plasma drug concentration at any time after administration can be calculated using the equations below.

$$C = Ae^{-\alpha t} + Be^{-\beta t} \tag{3.18}$$

$$n = \frac{t}{t_{1/2\alpha}} \tag{3.43}$$

$$N = \frac{t}{t_{1/2\beta}} \tag{3.44}$$

$$C = \frac{A}{2^n} + \frac{B}{2^N} \tag{3.45}$$

If $N \leq 0.1$ then the simplified form of equation 3.45 may be used, equation 3.46.

$$C = \frac{A}{2^n} + B \tag{3.46}$$

Drug elimination during distribution phase

One fact should be carefully noted by the reader wishing to calculate changes of plasma drug concentration during the distribution phase of drug kinetics. Drug (re)distribution from the central compartment volume to the whole of the distribution volume of that drug is the main reason, but not the only reason that plasma drug concentration falls rapidly during the distribution phase. Drug elimination also occurs during the distribution phase, as clearance of drugs during this phase is the same as during the elimination phase. A significant proportion of a given dose of a drug may actually be eliminated during the distribution phase, if the duration of the distribution phase of that drug is a significant fraction of the elimination half life, e.g. as for pancuronium or midazolam. This means that the values of "n" and "N" should always be calculated when using equation 3.46 to see if the conditions under which this equation can be used are satisfied.

EXAMPLE 5.1:

If the duration of the distribution phase of a drug is a significant fraction of the elimination half life of that drug, a significant proportion of that drug may actually be eliminated during the distribution phase. This is well illustrated by the example of pancuronium.

What fraction of a given intravenous bolus dose of pancuronium is eliminated during the DISTRIBUTION phase?

Elimination of pancuronium is described using a monoexponential decay equation. Such an equation can be used to calculate the fraction of a single dose of pancuronium eliminated during the distribution phase. The equation for a monoexponential decay process has been discussed in chapters 1 and 3 [see equations 1.9 and 3.12]. Let X_0 be the amount of drug present in the body at time = 0, and let "X_t" be the amount of drug in the body after time = "t" minutes has elapsed. The elimination rate constant β has its' usual meaning. Equation 5.1 then describes the amount of drug remaining in the body after a given time has elapsed.

$$X_t = X_0.e^{-\beta t} \qquad (5.1)$$

- Let $X_0 = 1$ so X_t is then automatically expressed as a fraction of X_0.
- Value of β for pancuronium = 0.0061 min^{-1}.
- Pancuronium $t_{1/2\alpha}$ = 10.7 minutes.
- Duration of pancuronium distribution phase = $4 \times t_{1/2\alpha} = 4 \times 10.7 = 42.8$ minutes.
- Substitute these values into equation 5.1 to get the fraction of the dose remaining in the body at the end of the distribution phase = $X_t = X_0.e^{-\beta t}$ = $1 \times e^{-0.0061 \times 42.8} = 0.77$.

-    This means that 0.23 = 23% of a bolus dose is eliminated during the distribution phase. This is a significant fraction of the administered dose.

Elimination phase

This is the phase in the concentration-time curve resulting from intravenous bolus administration of a drug when the drug concentration is declining at its' slowest rate. At this time the drug is fully distributed throughout its' distribution volume, and so no more (re)distribution occurs. The rate of decline of plasma drug concentration during the elimination phase is determined by the rate of drug elimination from the body.

Elimination phase plasma drug concentrations can be calculated using equations 3.18, 3.40 or 3.45. Equation 3.47 can be used to calculate plasma drug concentrations during the elimination phase when $n > 4$. However, equation 3.47 can only be applied when $n > 4$, otherwise the term $A/2^n$ is still significant and must be included in the calculation.

$$C = \frac{B}{2^N} \tag{3.47}$$

CONCENTRATION-EFFECT RELATIONSHIP

The plasma concentration of a drug administered as an intravenous bolus continuously changes. This means that effect compartment drug concentration cannot be readily calculated using a simple formula. There are two methods of calculating effect compartment drug concentrations in this situation.

- Use the series of differential equations, 3.48, 3.49 and 3.50, which describe the effect compartment model shown in figure 4.8

- A simpler method is to use the fact that the kinetics of the drug under consideration can readily be described with a 2-compartment model. This means that plasma drug concentrations can be calculated with equations 3.18, 3.40 or 3.45. Calculate the plasma concentrations at small time intervals and use Euler's method together with equation 4.10 to calculate effect compartment drug concentrations. This method has been discussed at the end of chapter 4, and is used throughout this chapter.

However, neither of the above methods can be used in clinical practice. All that can be done is to list some guidelines relating plasma to effect compartment drug concentrations. These guidelines all relate plasma drug concentration to the MEC for a given effect due to the drug under consideration.

- Plasma drug concentrations must be equal to, or greater than the MEC of a given effect due to that drug if the drug is to exert that effect.

- If **A** + **B**, but not **B** alone is greater than the MEC, any clinically significant effect of that drug will be terminated relatively rapidly by drug redistribution.

- If **B** alone is greater than the MEC, any clinically significant effect of the drug will be mainly terminated by drug elimination.

- If the plasma drug concentration is constant or changes only slowly, both plasma and effect compartment concentrations may be considered to be approximately equal.

- In situations where the plasma drug concentration is INCREASING rapidly, effect compartment concentration of the drug is always less than that in the plasma. This means that the clinically significant effect due to the drug will occur when the plasma drug concentration is greater than the MEC of that drug. The reverse occurs when the plasma concentration of a drug is rapidly decreasing.

Most examples in this chapter are accompanied by a figure in which effect compartment and plasma drug concentrations are shown simultaneously. These figures demonstrate one or more of the above points.

Application of methods

The use of the equations and concentration-effect relationship described in the preceding pages are able to be made evident to the reader with an example, example 5.2.

EXAMPLE 5.2:

The plasma concentration of a non-depolarizing muscle relaxant must at least be equal to the EC_{80} for the relaxant under consideration if a surgeon is to easily perform intra-abdominal surgery [see appendix-A for explanation of the EC_{80}]. How long will such a degree of muscle relaxation be provided by a single 0.1 mg/kg intravenous bolus dose of pancuronium?

- $t_{1/2\alpha}$ = 10.7 min.
- $t_{1/2\beta}$ = 114 min.
- MEC for muscle relaxation sufficient for intra-abdominal surgery = the EC_{80} = 0.27 mg/L for pancuronium.
- A = dose x A_x = 0.1 x 5.54 = 0.554 mg/L.
- B = dose x B_x = 0.1 x 2.8 = 0.28 mg/L.
- The value of B is very close to that for the EC_{80}. This makes it likely that the plasma and effect compartment pancuronium concentrations will fall

below the EC_{80} by the time that the distribution phase is complete. Pancuronium concentrations will now be calculated using the equations listed in this section. The change of plasma and effect compartment pancuronium concentrations with time are shown in figure 5.1.

At time = 0 min, C = A + B = 0.554 + 0.28 = 0.834 mg/L.

After 1 x $t_{1/2\alpha}$ = 10.7 minutes.
- n = 1.
- N = 10.7/114 = 0.094. As N < 0.1, this means that equation 3.46 may be used.
- $C = B + A/2^n$ = 0.28 + 0.554/2 = 0.28 + 0.277 = 0.56 mg/L.

After 2 x $t_{1/2\alpha}$ = 21.4 minutes.
- n = 2.
- N = 21.4/114 = 0.188. N > 0.1, and so use equation 3.45.
- **Method 1:** $C = A/2^n + B/2^N = 0.554/2^2 + 0.28/2^{0.188}$ = 0.384 mg/L.
- **Method 2:** $C = 0.277/2 + 0.28/2^{0.188}$ = 0.14 + 0.246 = 0.386 mg/L.

After 3 x $t_{1/2\alpha}$ = 32.1 minutes.
- n = 3.
- N = 32.1/114 = 0.282. N > 0.1, and so use equation 3.45.
- **Method 1:** $C = A/2^n + B/2^N = 0.554/2^3 + 0.28/2^{0.282}$ = 0.3 mg/L.
- **Method 2:** $C = 0.14/2 + 0.28/2^{0.282}$ = 0.07 + 0.23 = 0.3 mg/L.

After 4 x $t_{1/2\alpha}$ = 42.8 minutes.
- n = 4.
- N = 42.8/114 = 0.375. N > 0.1, and so use equation 3.45.
- **Method 1:** $C = A/2^n + B/2^N = 0.554/2^4 + 0.28/2^{0.375}$ = 0.25 mg/L.
- **Method 2:** $C = 0.07/2 + 0.28/2^{0.375}$ = 0.25 mg/L.

Plasma and effect compartment pancuronium concentrations fall below the EC_{80} after a time approximately equal to 4 x $t_{1/2\alpha}$ = 42.8 minutes. Clinical experiment confirms that the time taken for muscle contraction strength to return to 25% of normal after such a dose of pancuronium is 35 ± 5 minutes [1]. This is also the duration of relaxation sufficient to permit intra-abdominal surgery. As was expected, the effective clinical action of pancuronium at this dose is terminated mainly by distribution, and to a lesser degree by elimination. These concentration changes are also shown in figure 5.1.

Equation 3.47 may be used to calculate the change in concentration with time during the elimination phase.

After 1 x $t_{1/2\beta}$ = 114 minutes.

- n = 114/10.7. As n > 4, use equation 3.47.
- N = 1.
- C = $B/2^N$ = 0.28/2 = 0.14 mg/L. This is far below the EC_{80}, and so this dose of pancuronium will certainly not be effective at this time.

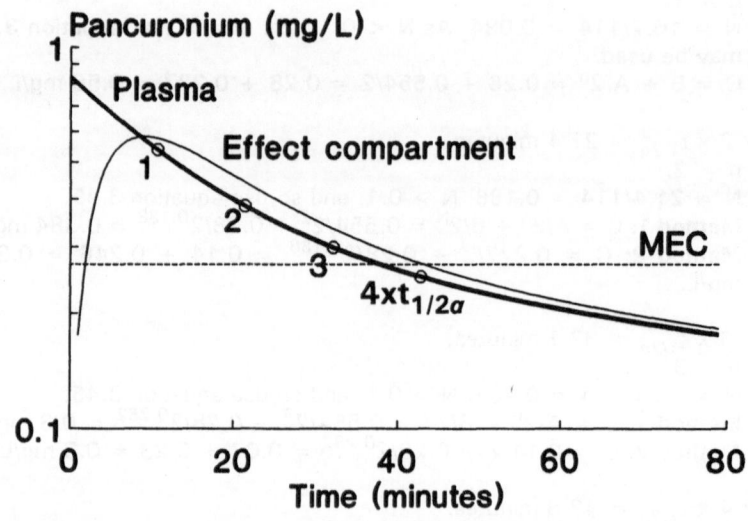

Figure 5.1: Plasma and effect compartment pancuronium concentrations resulting from a single bolus dose of 0.1 mg/kg. These are shown in relation to the MEC and multiples of the $t_{1/2\alpha}$.

These equations and methods may also be applied equally well to other common clinical problems and uses of anesthetic drugs.

INDUCTION AGENTS

Anesthetic induction agents present some interesting kinetic and dynamic problems. The pharmacological properties of these drugs are characterized by several features [see also table 5.1].

- They usually induce hypnosis together with loss of the eyelid reflex within 30-60 seconds after administration of an intravenous bolus dose.

- Drug concentrations sufficient to induce loss of consciousness, and to depress central nervous system reflexes to a depth sufficient to depress the eyelid reflex are only really achieved in the pre-recirculation and distribution phases of all the drugs listed in table 5.1. (Re)distribution of drug from the V_c to the whole of the V_d reduces plasma drug concentrations to levels far below the MEC for hypnosis. This means that drug elimination by either metabolism or excretion is **NOT** a factor which determines the speed of recovery after administration of these drugs.

- Because of the above, the duration of hypnosis induced by these drugs is of short duration. Consciousness usually returns spontaneously within 10-20 minutes.

Table 5.1.

Plasma drug concentrations resulting from the administration of the usual clinical doses of various anesthetic induction drugs. These are shown in relation to the MEC of each drug for various clinical effects.

Drug	MEC for hypnosis (mg/L)	MEC for eyelid reflex (mg/L)	MEC for myocardial depression (mg/L)	Dose (mg/kg)	C_{pr} (mg/L)	C_o = A+B (mg/L)	B (mg/L)
Thiopental	10	23^2	70^3	5	77^{10}	40	1.3
Methohexital	3.4	4.4^4	10^5	1.5	?	4.3	0.3
Ketamine	1	?	24^6	2	?	1.9	0.3
Etomidate	0.21	0.46^7	15^3	0.3	?	1	0.1
Propofol	1	?	10^8	2	50^9	4.1	0.3
Midazolam	0.2	?	15^{11}	0.15	?	1.6	0.06
Diazepam	0.96	?	20^{11}	0.3	?	1.4	0.2
Alfentanil	1.2	?	?	0.12	5^{12}	0.71	0.2

C_{pr} = peak pre-recirculation phase drug concentration. Drug concentrations in this phase are higher than the MEC's for hypnosis and myocardial depression.

C_0 = peak concentration calculated with 2-compartment model. Drug concentrations are sufficient to induce hypnosis with depression of the eyelid reflex, but not to induce myocardial depression.

B = theoretical maximum drug concentration after complete distribution has occurred. Concentrations are insufficient to induce hypnosis, depression of eyelid reflex or myocardial depression.

- Administration of these drugs in doses sufficient to induce rapid loss of consciousness and eyelid reflex is often associated with cardiovascular depression, as drug concentrations sufficient to cause cardiovascular depression are achieved in the pre-recirculation phase. This accounts for both the rapid onset, as well as the short duration of cardiovascular depression. Cardiovascular depression is often terminated by drug redistribution from the central blood volume to the V_c and V_d.

- Sometimes these drugs are used alone to provide anesthesia. Except for ketamine and alfentanil, none of the drugs used for intravenous induction of hypnosis possess any analgesic properties. Anesthesia with these drugs is due to induction of coma, a characteristic feature of which is a lack of any response to pain. Such a degree of central nervous system depression is also often associated with significant cardiovascular depression.

These kinetic and dynamic properties are able to be predicted to some extent using currently available data. Regrettably current kinetic data are deficient in one important area, the pre-recirculation phase, (i.e. 20-30 seconds after rapid intravenous injection). It is in this period that many of the induction agents exert an effect. However, despite this deficiency it is still possible to make some interesting predictions. Examples 5.3 and 5.4 demonstrate in more detail what has been discussed above and shown in table 5.1.

EXAMPLE 5.3:

Thiopental is one of the most commonly used intravenous induction agents in anesthesia. The usual dose is 3-6 mg/kg. Hypnosis together with loss of the eyelid reflex and cardiovascular depression are induced within 20-30 seconds after bolus administration of such a dose to the "average" adult patient into a vein in the dorsum of the hand, a forearm vein, or into a cubital fossa vein. Neither the speed of onset of hypnosis nor the occurrence of cardiovascular depression are well explained by current multicompartment pharmacokinetic models.

The arm-to-brain circulation time in the average adult is about 13-20 seconds. So thiopental will not even be present in the brain until this time has elapsed after intravenous bolus injection. Now hypnosis with loss of the eyelid reflex does occur by 20-30 seconds after intravenous bolus administration. Therefore the actual time available for thiopental to diffuse into, and induce hypnosis together with suppression of the eyelid reflex is only 7-17 seconds. This means that arterial blood thiopental concentrations must be quite high, otherwise the onset of sleep would not be so rapid. Such rapid transfer of thiopental across human cerebral capillaries does occur. Human experiment has shown that after injection of a bolus of thiopental into a cubital fossa vein, cerebral uptake is maximal 20 seconds after injection, and thiopental actually starts to diffuse out of the brain after 45 seconds [15,16].

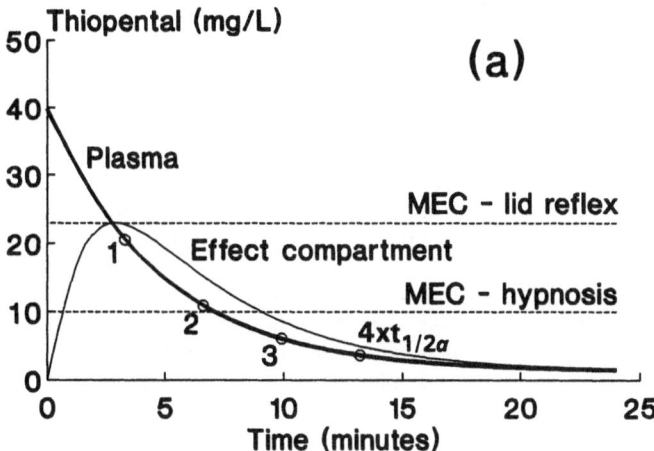

Figure 5.2: Plasma and CEREBRAL EFFECT COMPARTMENT concentrations resulting from a bolus injection of 5 mg/kg thiopental. Thiopental concentrations are shown in relation to the MEC for hypnosis, loss of lid reflex, and myocardial depression. The simulation in figure 5.2a uses a standard multicompartment model [parameters in appendix-A], while figure 5.2b uses a pre-recirculation phase physiological model [see chapter 2]. It is clear from figure 5.2a that a multicompartment model is unable to explain the clinical experience of all anesthesiologists that adults nearly always fall asleep within 30 seconds after such an intravenous bolus dose of thiopental. Figure 5.2b shows that a physiological model, used together with effect compartment modelling, can explain both the rapid onset of sleep and the myocardial depression observed.

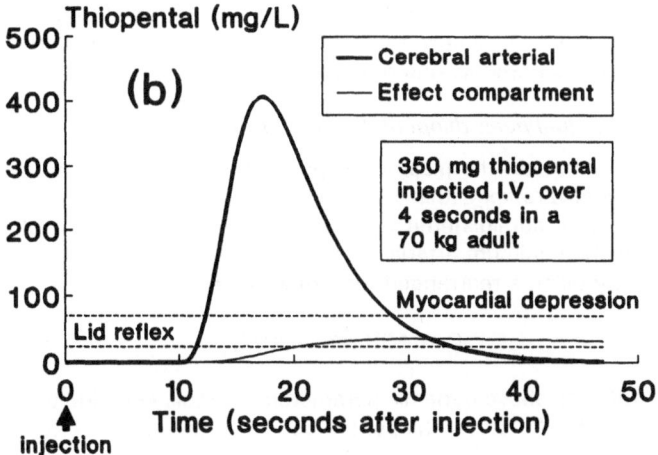

Consider a single rapid intravenous bolus dose of 5 mg/kg thiopental. What cerebral capillary blood thiopental concentrations are required to induce hypnosis in 20-30 seconds after injection? How long will hypnosis last? Will significant myocardial depression occur?

Data

- A bolus intravenous injection of thiopental is administered. Assume that hypnosis together with loss of the eyelid reflex is induced within 15 seconds = 0.25 minutes after arrival of thiopental in the cerebral circulation.
- MEC of thiopental for hypnosis = 10 mg/L [table 5.1].
- MEC of thiopental for loss of eyelid reflex = 23 mg/L [table 5.1].
- MEC of thiopental for myocardial depression = 70 mg/L [table 5.1].
- $t_{1/2}k_{eo}$ of thiopental = 1.2 minutes, and so k_{eo} = 0.693/1.2 = 0.5775 min^{-1}

Standard multicompartment kinetic-dynamic modelling

Figure 5.2 shows clearly that using kinetic data derived from intravenous plasma thiopental concentration-times curves, that only 50% of people will be asleep at one minute, and that it will take about three minutes before the eyelid reflex is lost in 50% of persons receiving a dose of 5 mg/kg. This is nonsense. Clinical experience with many tens of millions of patients shows that nearly all patients are asleep, and have lost their eyelid reflex within 20-30 seconds after intravenous bolus administration of such a dose of thiopental.

The main reason for such a gross discrepancy between theory and practice is deficient data. In this case, standard thiopental kinetic data as presented in appendix-A of this book, predict an initial plasma thiopental concentration which is simply too low, because data were derived from venous drug concentrations, and not arterial.

Calculation of actual peak thiopental concentration required

So how high must the plasma thiopental be if people are to fall asleep and lose their eyelid reflex within 15 seconds after administration of a 5mg/kg dose of thiopental administered as a single rapid intravenous bolus? The calculation of the minimum arterial plasma thiopental concentration required can be done by using a rearranged form of equation 4.14.

$$C = MEC/(1 - e^{-keo.t})$$

Substitute the above dynamic parameters into this equation to calculate the minimum steady state thiopental concentration needed to produce hypnosis with loss of eyelid reflex within 15 seconds.

$$C = MEC/(1 - e^{-keo.t}) = 23/(1 - e^{-0.5775 \times 0.25}) = 171.1 \text{ mg/L}.$$

Such a high thiopental concentration also readily explains the cardiovascular depression nearly always observed after bolus administration of such a dose of thiopental. It is well above the MEC for inducing myocardial depression.

A practical point can be added here too. Thiopental causes sleep and cardiovascular depression in one arm-to-brain circulation time, which is about 13-20 seconds [see table 2.1]. Now the first arteries that the thiopental enters after being pumped into the aorta, are the coronary arteries. These are situated just above the aortic valve. So after the first passage through the heart the myocardium is always initially perfused with blood containing a very high thiopental concentration.

The concentration calculated here is higher than reported pre-recirculation phase arterial thiopental concentrations. Peak arterial thiopental concentrations reported after administering 5 mg/kg over 30 seconds are never higher than 86 mg/L [10,14]. These measured concentrations are just sufficient to explain the observed central nervous system effects and the myocardial depression, but are unable to explain the rapidity of their onset. However there is a reason for the discrepancy. The reader should note that these reported measurements were made after infusing the thiopental induction dose of 5 mg/kg over 30 seconds. In clinical practice a thiopental dose of 5 mg/kg is usually administered over a period of 4-10 seconds, and not 30 seconds. This means that the peak pre-recirculation phase concentrations achieved in clinical practice are higher than those after a 30 second infusion of the same dose [see figure 5.2b for a simulation of a 5mg/kg dose injected over 4 seconds].

It is evident from this small example that the pre-recirculation phase kinetics of anesthetic induction agents is a topic which requires more study.

Duration of hypnosis

The duration of hypnosis resulting from a 5 mg/kg dose of thiopental lasts several minutes. This is far longer than the duration of the pre-recirculation phase, and so a multicompartment model is quite adequate to calculate the duration of hypnosis. The methods used are the same as for example 5.2 [see also fig 5.2].

- Thiopental dose = 5 mg/kg.
- MEC for hypnosis = 10 mg/L [appendix-A].
- $t_{1/2\alpha}$ = 3.3 minutes.
- $t_{1/2\beta}$ = 781 minutes.

- $A = \text{dose} \times A_x = 5 \times 7.68 = 38.4$ mg/L.
- $B = \text{dose} \times B_x = 5 \times 0.26 = 1.3$ mg/L.

At time = 0 minutes.
-    C = A + B = 38.4 + 1.3 = 39.7 mg/L.

At time = 1 x $t_{1/2\alpha}$ = 3.3 minutes.
-    n = 1
-    N = 3.3/781 < 0.1, so use equation 3.46. Even when n = 4, N < 0.1. So equation 3.46 can be used throughout the distribution period. Use method 2 from example 5.1.
-    C = B + A/2^n = 1.3 + 38.4/2 = 1.3 + 19.2 = 20.5 mg/L.

At time = 2 x $t_{1/2\alpha}$ = 2 x 3.3 = 6.6 minutes.
-    n = 2.
-    C = B + A/2^n = 1.3 + 19.2/2 = 1.3 + 9.6 = 10.9 mg/L.

At time = 3 x $t_{1/2\alpha}$ = 3 x 3.3 = 9.9 minutes.
-    n = 3.
-    C = B + A/2^n = 1.3 + 9.6/2 = 1.3 + 4.8 = 6.1 mg/L.

These calculations show that plasma and effect compartment thiopental concentrations fall below the MEC for hypnosis 6.5-10 minutes after intravenous bolus injection of a 5 mg/kg dose [see also figure 5.2]. This corresponds with the duration of hypnosis that is experimentally found for a 3.5-5.5 mg/kg dose of thiopental [13]. The hypnotic effect of such a dose of thiopental is so short that is terminated by (re)distribution rather than by drug elimination.

EXAMPLE 5.4:

Calculate the likely duration of hypnosis, and estimate the likelihood of myocardial depression resulting from an intravenous bolus dose of 0.3 mg/kg of etomidate.

-    MEC of etomidate for hypnosis = 0.21 mg/L [appendix-A].
-    MEC of etomidate for loss of eyelid reflex = 0.46 mg/L [table 5.1].
-    MEC of etomidate for myocardial depression = 15 mg/L [table 5.1].
-    $t_{1/2\alpha}$ = 2.6 minutes.
-    $t_{1/2\beta}$ = 67 minutes.

-    A = dose x A_x = 0.3 x 3 = 0.9 mg/L.
-    B = dose x B_x = 0.3 x 0.33 = 0.099 mg/L

At time = 0 minutes.
-    C = A + B = 0.9 + 0.099 = 1 mg/L.
-    This concentration is sufficient to induce hypnosis together with loss of the eyelid reflex, but insufficient to induce myocardial depression.

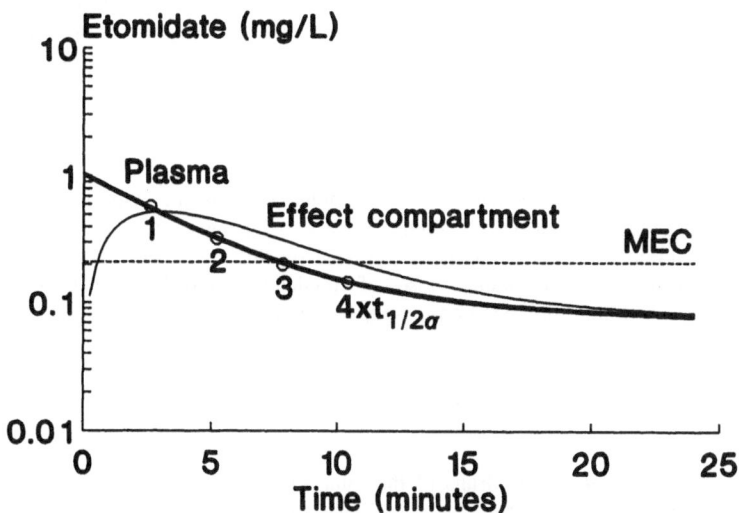

Figure 5.3: Plasma and effect compartment etomidate concentrations resulting from bolus administration of 0.3 mg/kg etomidate. These curves are shown in relation to the MEC for hypnosis and multiples of the $t_{1/2\alpha}$ of etomidate.

At time $= 1 \times t_{1/2\alpha} = 2.6$ minutes.
- $n = 1$.
- $N = 2.6/67 = 0.04$. As $N < 0.1$, use equation 3.46.
- $C = B + A/2^n = 0.099 + 0.9/2 = 0.099 + 0.45 = 0.55$ mg/L.
- As C is $>$ MEC for hypnosis and loss of eyelid reflex, the patient remains asleep.

At time $= 2 \times t_{1/2\alpha} = 2 \times 2.6 = 5.2$ minutes.
- $n = 2$.
- $N = 5.2/67 = 0.08$. As $N < 0.1$, use equation 3.46.
- $C = B + A/2^n = 0.099 + 0.45/2 = 0.099 + 0.225 = 0.324$ mg/L.
- As C is $>$ MEC for hypnosis, the patient remains asleep at this time.

At time $= 3 \times t_{1/2\alpha} = 3 \times 2.6 = 7.8$ minutes.
- $n = 3$.
- $N = 7.8/67 = 0.12$. As N is > 0.1, equation 3.40 must be used.
- $C = A/2^n + B/2^N = 0.225/2 + 0.099/2^{0.12} = 0.113 + 0.091 = 0.204$ mg/L.

- C is now = MEC for hypnosis. It is likely that the effect compartment etomidate concentration will fall below that required for hypnosis soon after this time [see also figure 5.3]. Figure 5.3 also shows that it takes about 10 minutes for the effect compartment etomidate concentration to fall below the MEC for hypnosis.

The duration of hypnosis calculated in this example corresponds with the experimentally determined hypnosis duration of 10-14 minutes for a 0.2-0.4 mg/kg intravenous bolus dose of etomidate [17]. Another feature of etomidate revealed by this calculation and table 5.1 is that cardiovascular depression due to clinical doses of etomidate is only likely to occur in the pre-recirculation phase, or after administration of very high doses.

USE OF ELIMINATION & DISTRIBUTION PHASES

It is common practice to divide drugs of the same group into "short-", "intermediate-" and "long-acting" drugs. This is actually a very arbitrary empirical division which actually has no pharmacokinetic or pharmacodynamic basis. Duration of drug effect is a function of factors such as $t_{1/2\alpha}$, $t_{1/2\beta}$, concentration-effect curve slope, and the dose administered. The effect of concentration-effect curve slope on drug dynamics has already been discussed in chapter 4, and so will not be repeated here. This section discusses the influence of drug kinetics on duration of drug effect.

Elimination half life and duration of effect

The effect duration of a drug is not necessarily directly proportional to the elimination half life of the drug. In fact a drug with a relatively short elimination half life may actually have a longer effect duration than a drug with a very much longer elimination half life. This is demonstrated in example 5.5 for morphine and methadone.

EXAMPLE 5.5:

Morphine and methadone are both opiates which are used to provide postoperative analgesia. The usual doses of both drugs for postoperative analgesia are the same, being 0.15 mg/kg. However the duration of postoperative analgesia due to a single intravenous dose of 0.15 mg/kg methadone is shorter than that due to the same dose of morphine. The reasons for this are shown in this example, [see also figure 5.4].

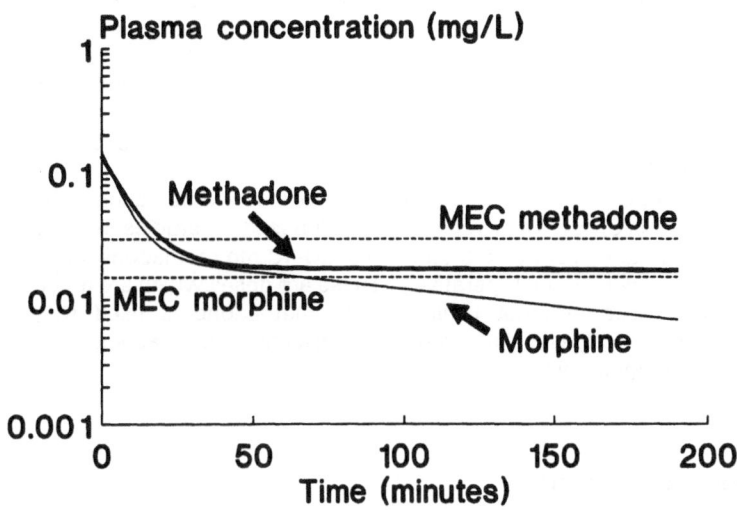

Figure 5.4: Plasma concentration-time curves of intravenous bolus doses of 0.15 mg/kg methadone and morphine in "average" adult patients. These curves are shown in relationship to the MEC for postoperative analgesia of each drug.

	Morphine	Methadone
Dose (mg/kg)	0.15	0.15
MEC (analgesia) (mg/L)	0.015	0.03
$t_{1/2\alpha}$ (minutes)	4.4	6.1
$t_{1/2\beta}$ (minutes)	111	2100
A_x (kg/L)	0.84	0.79
B_x (kg/L)	0.15	0.12
$A = \text{dose} \times A_x$ (mg/L)	0.126	0.119
$B = \text{dose} \times B_x$ (mg/L)	0.023	0.018

Time	n	N	Concn. (mg/L)	n	N	Concn. (mg/L)
$0 \times t_{1/2\alpha}$	0	0	0.15	0	0	0.14
$1 \times t_{1/2\alpha}$	1	0.04	0.09	1	0.003	0.08
$2 \times t_{1/2\alpha}$	2	0.08	0.05	2	0.006	0.05
$3 \times t_{1/2\alpha}$	3	0.12	0.04	3	0.009	0.03
$4 \times t_{1/2\alpha}$	4	0.16	0.03	4	0.012	0.025 < MEC
$1 \times t_{1/2\beta}$	25.2	1	0.01 < MEC	344	1	0.01 < MEC

It is apparent from these calculations that the duration of analgesia due to methadone is considerably shorter than that due to morphine. The clinical effect of methadone is terminated by distribution, while the effect of an identical dose of morphine is terminated by elimination. This difference is the result of a different dose-to-MEC relationship for these two drugs. One conclusion from this is that a dose of 0.15 mg/kg methadone is too low for the purpose for which it is used.

Prolonged postoperative analgesia with methadone has been reported by Gourlay et al [18,19]. Their reports were all based on studies in which adult patients were administered a total dose of 20-40 mg methadone intraoperatively and immediately postoperatively. These are doses which are much higher than those used in most clinics where methadone is used to provide postoperative analgesia. However it is certainly true that such doses do provide prolonged postoperative analgesia.

Dose and duration of drug effect

Example 5.5 demonstrated that dose is an important determinant of duration of drug effect. This is merely a restatement of what all clinicians know. The duration of drug effect is directly proportional to the drug dose. This is a principle which is applicable to all drugs. Examples 5.6 and 5.7 apply this principle to fentanyl and tubocurarine.

EXAMPLE 5.6:

Fentanyl is a drug which is either "short-" or "long-acting", depending on the dose administered. Consider two different intravenous bolus doses of fentanyl. A dose of 150 μg/70 kg (= 0.15 mg for an average adult), and one of 400 μg/70 kg (= 0.4 mg for an average adult).

- MEC for postoperative analgesia = 1 μg/L [appendix-A].
- $t_{1/2\alpha}$ = 9 minutes.
- $t_{1/2\beta}$ = 263 minutes.
- A_x = 1.09 kg/L
- B_x = 0.21 kg/L

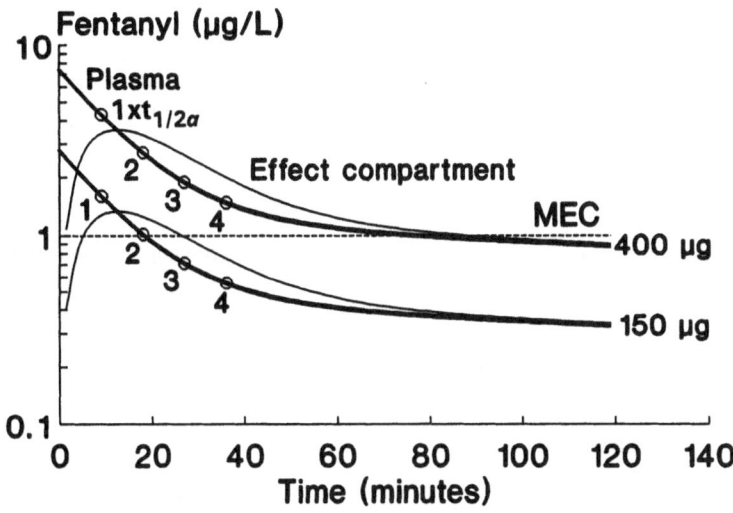

Figure 5.5: The changes of plasma and effect compartment concentrations with time after a dose of 150 μg/70 kg (= 0.15 mg for an adult), and another of 400 μg/70 kg (= 0.4 mg for an adult). The effect of the lower dose on postoperative analgesia is mainly terminated by distribution, while that of the higher dose by both distribution and elimination.

Dose			150 μg/70 kg	400 μg/70 kg
A = dose x A_x (μg/L)			2.34	6.23
B = dose x B_x (μg/L)			0.45	1.2
Time	n	N	Concn. (μg/L)	Concn. (μg/L)
$0 \times t_{1/2\alpha}$ = 0 min	0	0	2.81	7.42
$1 \times t_{1/2\alpha}$ = 9 min	1	0.034	1.61	4.28
$2 \times t_{1/2\alpha}$ = 18 min	2	0.068	1.01	2.7
$3 \times t_{1/2\alpha}$ = 27 min	3	0.1	0.71 < MEC	1.9
$4 \times t_{1/2\alpha}$ = 36 min	4	0.14	0.55 < MEC	1.47
$1 \times t_{1/2\beta}$ = 263 min	29.2	1	0.23 < MEC	0.6 < MEC

The plasma and effect compartment concentration of fentanyl is reduced below that required for postoperative analgesia by (re)distribution alone in the case of the dose of 150 μg/70 kg. However in the case of the larger 400 μg/70 kg dose, (re)distribution alone is not sufficient to reduce the plasma and effect compartment fentanyl concentration below that required for postoperative analgesia. In the latter situation, elimination of fentanyl is also required. Elimination is a much slower process than distribution, and so the plasma fentanyl concentration remains above the MEC for much longer [see figure 5.5].

This example shows that drug dose is an important factor determining duration of drug action.

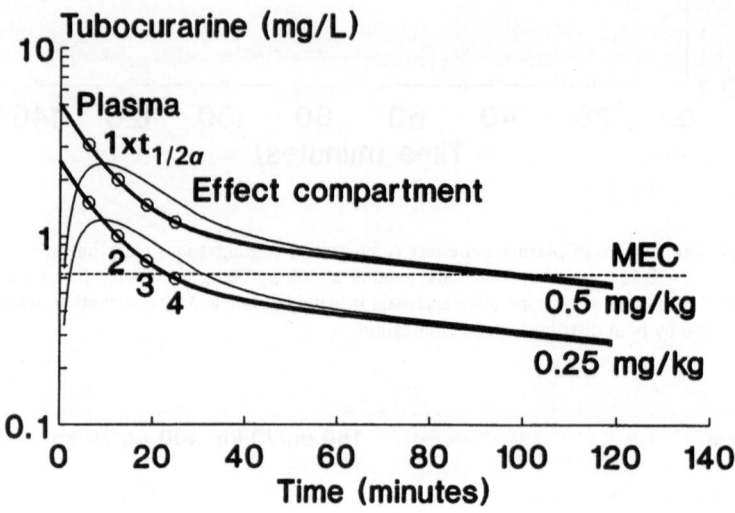

Figure 5.6: The change of plasma and effect compartment tubocurarine concentrations with time after administration of bolus intravenous doses of 0.25 mg/kg and 0.5 mg/kg. The curves are shown in relation to the MEC = EC_{80} and $t_{1/2\alpha}$ of tubocurarine.

EXAMPLE 5.7:

Another good example of the influence of dose on the duration of drug effect is also provided by the non-depolarizing muscle relaxants. Consider two different doses of tubocurarine, one of 0.25 mg/kg and one of 0.5 mg/kg.

- MEC $= EC_{80} = 0.63$ mg/L.
- $t_{1/2\alpha} = 6.2$ minutes.
- $t_{1/2\beta} = 119$ minutes.
- $A_x = 7.82$ kg/L
- $B_x = 2.18$ kg/L

Dose			0.25 (mg/kg)	0.5 (mg/kg)
$A =$ dose x A_x (mg/L)			1.96	3.91
$B =$ dose x B_x (mg/L)			0.55	1.09

Time	n	N	Concn. (mg/L)	Concn. (mg/L)
$0 \times t_{1/2\alpha} = 0$ min	0	0	2.5	5
$1 \times t_{1/2\alpha} = 6.2$ min	1	0.052	1.5	3
$2 \times t_{1/2\alpha} = 12.4$ min	2	0.104	1	2
$3 \times t_{1/2\alpha} = 18.6$ min	3	0.156	0.73	1.5
$4 \times t_{1/2\alpha} = 24.8$ min	4	0.208	0.6 < MEC	1.2
$1 \times t_{1/2\beta} = 119$ min	19.19	1	0.27 < MEC	0.55 < MEC

This example also demonstrates the same features demonstrated in example 5.6. Duration of drug effect, and whether that effect is terminated by distribution or elimination, is directly related to drug dose, [see also figure 5.6].

Another example of the same type as examples 5.6 and 5.7 is provided by the plasma- and effect compartment concentration-time curves of 0.05 mg/kg and 0.1 mg/kg pancuronium as shown in figures 4.13 and 5.1. This principle is applicable to all drugs, and not only the drugs used in anesthesia.

- Duration of drug effect is relatively **SHORT** if a dose is administered such that the effect compartment concentration is reduced below the MEC for that drug by **(re)distribution** rather than by **elimination**.

- Duration of drug effect is relatively **LONG** if a dose is administered such that the effect compartment concentration of that drug is reduced below the MEC for that drug by **elimination** rather than by **(re)distribution**.

CALCULATION OF DRUG DOSE

Equations 3.40 or 3.45 can be rearranged to make equations 5.2 and 5.3. These may be used to calculate drug dose.

$$\text{Dose} = \frac{C}{A_x e^{-\alpha t} + B_x e^{-\beta t}} \tag{5.2}$$

$$\text{Dose} = \frac{C}{A_x / 2^n + B_x / 2^N} \tag{5.3}$$

There are a number of useful applications for these equations.

• Doses of drugs which cause significant cardiovascular or respiratory depression should be kept as low as possible while still being effective. A drug dose can be calculated such that minimum dose required for an effect is administered. This will minimize the magnitude of any drug concentration related undesirable effects.

• Some patients have hepatic insufficiency, renal failure, cardiac failure, or any combination of one or more disorders which retard drug elimination. Yet these same patients may require drugs whose elimination is retarded by these disorders. These patients should be administered doses of these drugs such that the termination of drug effect is by distribution rather than elimination.

• Drug doses may be calculated such that a given plasma concentration of a drug is present at any desired time. This is useful during anesthesia. If the duration of a surgical procedure is known, drug doses may be calculated so the effects of the drugs administered are terminated spontaneously by the processes of distribution and elimination by the end of the operation.

EXAMPLE 5.8:

A female patient is scheduled to undergo a laparoscopy under general anaesthesia for sterilization by means of clipping the fallopian tubes. The procedure will last about 15 minutes. As the patient is not anxious, and is to be discharged from the hospital at the end of the day, she receives no sedative premedication. After induction, anesthesia is to be maintained with a non-depolarizing muscle relaxant, together with alfentanil and 66% nitrous oxide to provide both analgesia and hypnosis. Calculate a dose of alfentanil to be administered at the start of the operation sufficient to satisfy the following criteria [see figure 5.7].

1. The intraoperative plasma alfentanil concentration must be high enough, when supplemented with nitrous oxide, to provide analgesia for the surgical procedure performed.
2. The plasma alfentanil concentration at the end of the operation will not cause significant respiratory depression.
3. The plasma alfentanil concentration at the end of operation is sufficient to provide some postoperative analgesia.

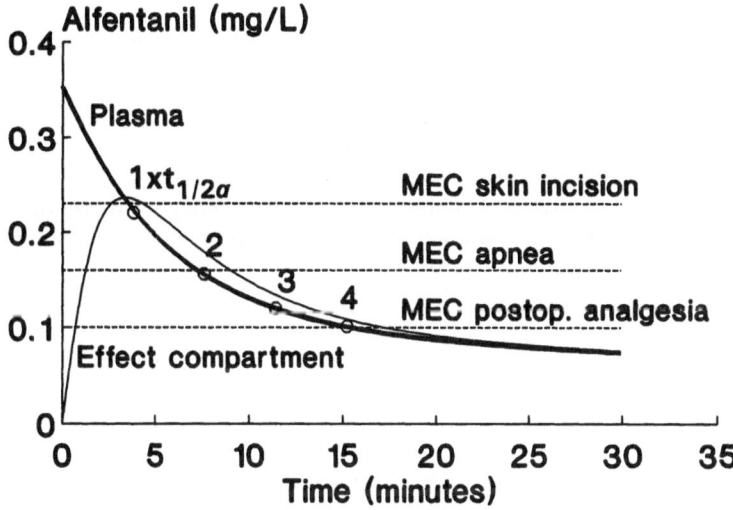

Figure 5.7: The effect compartment and plasma concentration-time curves of alfentanil resulting from a single bolus dose of 0.06 mg/kg (= 4.2 mg for a 70 kg adult), are shown in relation to the MEC values of alfentanil for skin incision, postoperative analgesia, and respiratory depression. The calculations required are demonstrated in example 5.8.

Parameters

-   Duration of surgical procedure = t = 15 minutes.
-   MEC of alfentanil for skin incision when supplemented with nitrous oxide = 0.23 mg/L [20]
-   MEC of alfentanil for apnea when 66% N_2O is administered = 0.16 mg/L [21].

- MEC of alfentanil for postoperative analgesia = 0.1 mg/L [appendix-A].
- Let the desired plasma concentration after 15 minutes be = C = 0.1 mg/L. This is a concentration which will permit adequate spontaneous respiration, yet is sufficient to provide postoperative analgesia.

Calculate dose

- $t_{1/2\alpha}$ = 3.8 minutes, and so at 15 minutes n = $t/t_{1/2\alpha}$ = 15/3.8 = 3.95.
- $t_{1/2\beta}$ = 70 minutes, and so at 15 minutes N = $t/t_{1/2\beta}$ = 15/70 = 0.21.
- A_x = 4.24 kg/L.
- B_x = 1.64 kg/L.
- Substitute these values into equation 5.3 to get the dose required to satisfy the above three criteria.

Dose = $C/(A_x/2^n + B_x/2^N)$ = $0.1/(4.24/2^{3.95} + 1.64/2^{0.21})$ = 0.06 mg/kg.

So for the "average" 70 kg adult this means a dose of 4.2 mg alfentanil. Such a dose of alfentanil is not unusual during laparoscopy in an unpremedicated patient who receives no anesthetic vapor to supplement the analgesic effects of alfentanil and nitrous oxide.

EXAMPLE 5.9:

Non-depolarizing muscle relaxants are mainly eliminated by the liver, kidneys, or both. Some patients with renal and or hepatic dysfunction undergo surgery. A non-depolarizing muscle relaxant is frequently administered during anesthesia. The main concern of the anesthesiologist administering these drugs to such patients is to avoid prolonged muscle relaxation because of reduced drug elimination.

Prolonged muscle relaxation can be avoided by administering doses of non-depolarizing relaxants which will provide effective plasma drug concentrations only during the distribution phase. Distribution will then terminate clinically useful muscle relaxant activity. Drug distribution is a process which has nothing to do with drug metabolism or excretion, and still occurs even when a drug is unable to be eliminated.

Calculate doses of various non-depolarizing muscle relaxants such that their effect is terminated by distribution in a time equal to 3 x $t_{1/2\alpha}$.

Assumptions for dose calculation

- In the case of the non-depolarizing muscle relaxants, the MEC at which intra-abdominal surgery is just possible, and at which the relaxant effect is easily antagonized is the EC_{80} [see appendix-A]. Therefore a muscle relaxant concentration greater than, or equal to the EC_{80} is defined as an effective drug concentration.

- Assume that absolutely no elimination of an administered muscle relaxant occurs. This means that the elimination half life of each non-depolarizing muscle relaxant is infinitely long.
- Let the duration of the period during which plasma muscle relaxant concentration is greater than the EC_{80} be equal to $3 \times t_{1/2\alpha}$.
- Set the muscle relaxant concentration equal to the EC_{80} at time = $3 \times t_{1/2\alpha}$.

Calculation of dose

An infinitely long elimination half life means $\beta = 0$ and $N = 0$. So $1/2^N = 1/2^0 = 1$. This means that equation 3.46 can be used to calculate the dose required.

$$C = Dose(B + A/2^n) \tag{3.46}$$

Substitute EC_{80} for "C", and let n = 3. This yields the formula required to calculate a dose satisfying the above requirements.

$$Dose = \frac{EC_{80}}{(B + A/2^3)} = \frac{EC_{80}}{(B + A/8)}$$

The above formula has been used to construct table 5.2.

Table 5.2.
Doses of non-depolarizing muscle relaxants which have a clinical effect duration of $3 \times t_{1/2\alpha}$, when administered as intravenous bolus doses to HEALTHY NORMAL adults.

Drug	EC_{80} (mg/L)	Dose (mg/kg)	Theoretical effect duration $= 3 \times t_{1/2\alpha}$ (minutes)
Gallamine	7.2	1.46	20.1
Tubocurarine	0.63	0.2	18.6
Alcuronium	0.66	0.23	41.4
Pancuronium	0.27	0.08	32.1
Vecuronium	0.15	0.063	22.5

REPEAT DOSES

Repeat doses of drugs are often administered during most anesthetics. Inappropriately timed, or excessively large repeat doses are often the cause of problems with induced or spontaneous reversal of anesthetic drug effect. This section provides a method of analyzing the kinetics and dynamics of repeat drug doses.

Calculation of new "A" and "B"

The magnitudes of the variables "A" and "B" are reduced by the processes of distribution and elimination respectively. After a given time "t" subsequent to intravenous bolus drug administration, the magnitudes of "A" and "B" are given by equations 5.4 and 5.5.

$$A_{(at\ time\ =\ t)} = A_{(at\ time\ =\ 0)} \cdot e^{-\alpha t} \qquad (5.4)$$

$$B_{(at\ time\ =\ t)} = B_{(at\ time\ =\ 0)} \cdot e^{-\beta t} \qquad (5.5)$$

If a second drug dose is administered, the new values of "A" and "B" are the sum of the values resulting from the repeat drug dose, and the remainder of the previous drug dose. This is shown by equations 5.6 and 5.7.

$$A = A_R + A_p.e^{-\alpha t} \qquad (5.6)$$

$$B = B_R + B_p.e^{-\beta t} \qquad (5.7)$$

P is a subscript indicating that the value of that parameter is from the previous drug dose.
R is a subscript indicating that the value of that parameter is from the repeat drug dose.
A and **B** have their usual meanings.

Calculation of drug concentration

After calculation of the new values of "A" and "B", drug concentrations at any time after administration of the repeat dose are calculated using equation 3.18, 3.40 or 3.45.

EXAMPLE 5.10:

Pancuronium is one of the most popular non-depolarizing neuromuscular blocking drugs. The usual initial bolus dose administered to adults is 4 mg, and 1 mg is the repeat bolus dose. The changes of plasma drug concentration with time as a result of administering an initial 4 mg bolus dose followed by a 1 mg repeat bolus will now be calculated.

- MEC = 0.27 mg/L.
- $t_{1/2\alpha}$ = 10.7 minutes.
- $t_{1/2\beta}$ = 114 minutes.
- A_x = 5.54 kg/L.
- B_x = 2.8 kg/L.

Initial dose

- Dose = 4 mg/70 kg = 0.057 mg/kg.
- A = dose x A_x = 0.057 x 5.54 = 0.32 mg/L.
- B = dose x B_x = 0.057 x 2.8 = 0.16 mg/L.

At time = 0 minutes.
- C = A + B = 0.32 + 0.16 = 0.48 mg/L.

At time = 1 x $t_{1/2\alpha}$ = 10.7 minutes.
- n = 1.
- N = 10.7/114 = 0.094.
- C = $A/2^n$ + $B/2^N$ = 0.32/2 + 0.16/1.06 = 0.16 + 0.15 = 0.31 mg/L.

At time = 2 x $t_{1/2\alpha}$ = 2 x 10.7 = 21.4 minutes.
- n = 2.
- N = 21.4/114 = 0.19.
- C = $A/2^n$ + $B/2^N$ = 0.32/4 + 0.16/1.14 = 0.08 + 0.14 = 0.22 mg/L.

- This concentration is less than the MEC, and a repeat dose is required.

First repeat dose

- Repeat dose = 1 mg/70 kg = 0.014 mg/kg.
  A_R = dose x A_x = 0.014 x 5.54 = 0.078 mg/L.
  B_R = dose x B_x = 0.014 x 2.8 = 0.04 mg/L.

- Repeat dose administered at a time = 21.4 minutes = 2 x $t_{1/2\alpha}$ after initial dose of 0.057 mg/kg. So new values of "A" and "B" after repeat dose are;

  A = A_R + $A_P/2^n$ = 0.078 + 0.32/2^2 = 0.078 + 0.08 = 0.158 mg/L
  B = B_R + $B_P/2^N$ = 0.04 + 0.16/$2^{0.19}$ = 0.04 + 0.14 = 0.18 mg/L

At time = 0 after repeat dose.
- C = A + B = 0.158 + 0.18 = 0.338 mg/L.

At time = 1 x $t_{1/2\alpha}$ after repeat dose = 10.7 minutes.
- n = 1.
- N = 10.7/114 = 0.094.
- C = $A/2^n$ + $B/2^N$ = 0.158/2 + 0.18/1.06 = 0.08 + 0.17 = 0.25 mg/L.
- This plasma pancuronium concentration is less than the EC_{80}, and so a repeat dose is needed again at this time.

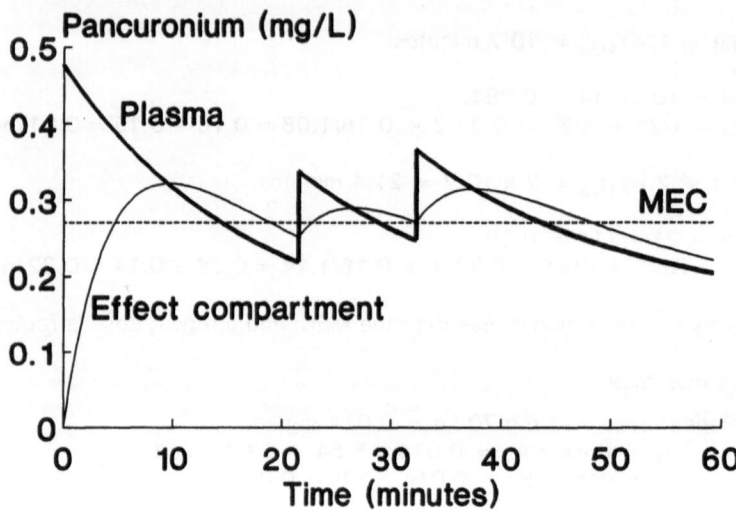

Figure 5.8: Plasma and effect compartment pancuronium concentration changes with time after administration of an initial 4 mg bolus dose followed by 2 repeat 1 mg bolus doses in an "average" 70 kg adult. These changes are shown in relation to the MEC = EC_{80}.

Second repeat dose

- Repeat dose = 1 mg/70 kg = 0.014 mg/kg.
    A_R = dose x A_x = 0.014 x 5.54 = 0.078 mg/L.
    B_R = dose x B_x = 0.014 x 2.8 = 0.04 mg/L.

- Second repeat dose is administered 10.7 minutes $= 1 \times t_{1/2\sigma}$ after first repeat dose. So the new values for "A" and "B" are;

$$A = A_R + A_P/2^n = 0.078 + 0.08 = 0.158 \text{ mg/L.}$$
$$B = B_R + B_P/2^N = 0.04 + 0.17 = 0.21 \text{ mg/L.}$$

At time $= 0$ after second repeat dose.
- $C = A + B = 0.158 + 0.21 = 0.368 \text{ mg/L.}$

At time $= 1 \times t_{1/2\sigma}$ after second repeat dose $= 10.7$ minutes.
- $n = 1$.
- $N = 10.7/114 = 0.094$.
- $C = A/2^n + B/2^N = 0.158/2 + 0.21/1.06 = 0.08 + 0.2 = 0.28 \text{ mg/L.}$

- This plasma concentration is very close to the MEC and so a repeat dose will be required soon after this time.

The procedure demonstrated in example 5.10 can be continued indefinitely for as many repeat doses as desired.

Single dose, or multiple smaller doses?

A given dose of a drug may either be administered as a single dose, or the dose may be divided into smaller doses. In clinical anesthetic practice it is often very practical to administer some drugs in small divided doses.

- In the case of non-depolarizing muscle relaxants this is a very practical dosing strategy. The reason for this is that while the duration of a given operation is predictable within certain limits, its duration is not always constant. A given drug dose can be administered as small doses given repeatedly as the need arises. The advantage of this is, that if the operation is ready sooner than expected, the effect of the muscle relaxant can be easily antagonized sooner than if a large single dose had been given. Example 5.11 gives an example of this.

- Opiates always cause respiratory depression if the plasma concentration is high enough. If a given dose of an opiate is administered as smaller divided doses, the chance of significant respiratory depression is reduced. This is demonstrated in example 5.12.

EXAMPLE 5.11:

There are two schools of thought with regard to administration of muscle relaxants. Proponents of one method administer frequent smaller doses, while proponents of the other school of thought administer fewer larger doses. For example, consider the administration of pancuronium to provide abdominal muscle relaxation for a procedure such as a cholecystectomy. This is a procedure which can last between 30-60 minutes.

Single, large dose method

A single dose of 0.1 mg/kg pancuronium, (about 7-8 mg in a normal adult), could be administered at the start of the operation. This would provide adequate muscle relaxation for about 40-45 minutes. At about 40-45 minutes the plasma and effect compartment pancuronium concentration would be equivalent to the EC_{80}. So any residual paralysis of the pancuronium would be easily be antagonized with the usual doses of atropine and an anticholinesterase. This dose is therefore a good choice for a surgeon who completes a cholecystectomy in this time. Example 5.2 shows the plasma concentration calculations for this, and figure 5.1 shows both the plasma and effect compartment pancuronium concentrations after such a dose of pancuronium.

The main problem presented with this dosage regimen is the rapid or unpredictable surgeon. A surgeon may finish the operation in 30 minutes. In that case the effects of the pancuronium would be more difficult to antagonize as the pancuronium concentration is much higher after 30 minutes than after 45 minutes.

Repeat doses are required if the operation lasts much longer than 40-45 minutes.

Multiple, lower dose method

Another method is to insert an endotracheal tube with the assistance of suxamethonium. Subsequently administer 0.05-0.06 mg/kg pancuronium, (about 4 mg for the average adult), and repeat doses of 0.0125-0.015 mg/kg, (about 1 mg for the average adult), as required. This has been shown in example 5.10 and figure 5.8.

Example 5.10 demonstrates that the total dose of pancuronium required for 40-45 minutes clinical muscle relaxation is only about 6 mg for the average adult when smaller doses are used. About 8 mg is required were the pancuronium to have all been administered as a single dose at the beginning of the operation. Such a method minimizes the total dose of muscle relaxant required per unit time. This is of importance in patients whose elimination of drugs such as muscle relaxants is impaired. Another advantage of the smaller dose method is also demonstrated by example 5.10. Repeat doses were required after 20 and 30 minutes. Were the surgeon to have finished by 20 or 30 minutes, reversal of the residual effects of the pancuronium would have been readily achieved at these times.

EXAMPLE 5.12:

Alfentanil is an ideal drug to provide analgesia for short surgical procedures. A common technique is to administer intermittent bolus doses of a hypnotic drug and alfentanil while letting the patient breathe spontaneously while receiving oxygen and nitrous oxide by face mask. If too much alfentanil is administered at any one time, apnea occurs, and the respiration must be assisted. During a short procedure such as abscess drainage, uterine curettage, cystoscopy, or a wound dressing, a total dose of 2.5 mg alfentanil may be administered to the average adult. Calculate the plasma alfentanil concentrations arising from a single bolus dose of 2.5 mg, or of five divided doses of 0.5 mg in an average 70 kg adult.

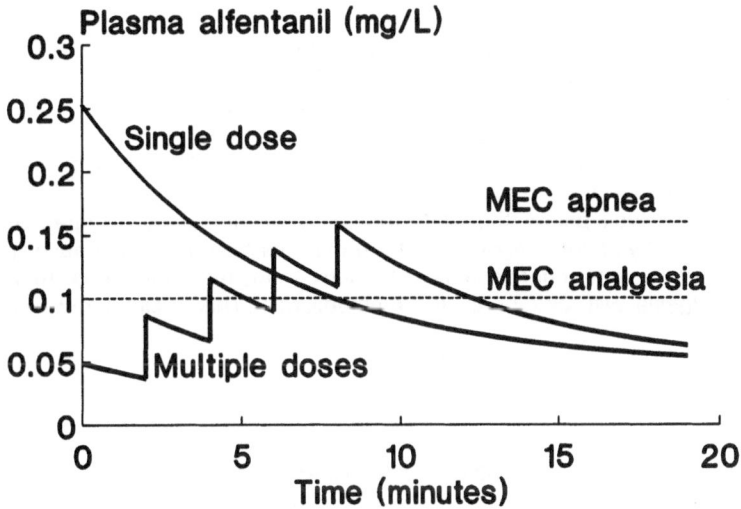

Figure 5.9: Plasma alfentanil concentration-time curves resulting from administration of either a large single bolus of 43 μg/kg (= 3 mg for an average adult), and of smaller intermittent boluses of 8.6 μg/kg (= 0.6 mg for an average adult), administered at two minute intervals. These curves are shown in relation to the MEC levels for apnea and postoperative analgesia.

Kinetic and dynamic parameters

- Alfentanil MEC to produce apnea = 0.16 mg/L [20].
- Alfentanil MEC to provide postoperative analgesia = 0.1 mg/L.
- A_x = 4.24 kg/L.
- B_x = 1.64 kg/L.

Single dose

-    3 mg alfentanil is administered as a single dose.
-    Dose = 3 mg/70 kg = 0.043 mg/kg.
-    A = dose x A_x = 0.043 x 4.24 = 0.182 mg/L.
-    B = dose x B_x = 0.043 x 1.64 = 0.071 mg/L.
-    Initial concentration after bolus dose = C_0 = A + B = 0.182 + 0.071 = 0.253 mg/L.
-    This alfentanil plasma concentration is likely to cause apnea as it is greater than the MEC for apnea.

Divided doses

-    5 doses of 0.6 mg = a total dose of 3 mg.
-    Dose = 0.6 mg/70 kg = 0.0086 mg/kg.
-    A = dose x A_x = 0.0086 x 4.24 = 0.036 mg/L.
-    B = dose x B_x = 0.0086 x 1.64 = 0.014 mg/L.
-    Initial concentration after a single bolus dose = C_0 = A + B = 0.036 + 0.014 = 0.05 mg/L.
-    This is well below the MEC for analgesia and apnea. Repeat doses spaced by an interval of at least 2-4 minutes are unlikely to cause apnea. However one consequence of such a dosing regimen is that any analgesia will take longer to be established. This is simulated in figure 5.9.

CONCLUDING REMARKS

This chapter presents a simplified approach to the application of pharmacokinetic and pharmacodynamic principles. However despite the simplicity of the methods demonstrated, they are capable of explaining most of the effects of intravenous drugs used in clinical anesthetic practice. The reader is encouraged to apply these methods to other problems encountered in clinical practice.

REFERENCES

1.   Fahey MR, et al: Clinical pharmacology of ORG NC45 (Norcuron"). A new nondepolarizing muscle relaxant. *Anesthesiology*, 1981: 55: 6-11.
2.   Becker KE: Plasma levels of thiopental necessary for anesthesia. *Anesthesiology*, 1978: 49: 192-196.
3.   Kissin I, et al: Inotropic and anesthetic potencies of etomidate and thiopental in dogs. *Anesthesia and Analgesia*, 1983: 62: 961-965.

4. Lauven PM, et al: Venous threshold concentrations of methohexitone. *Anesthesiology*, 1985: 63: A368.
5. Todd MM, et al: The hemodynamic consequences of high-dose methohexital anesthesia in humans. *Anesthesiology*, 1984: 61: 495-501.
6. Kaukinen S: The combined effects of antihypertensive drugs and anesthetics (Halothane and Ketamine) on the isolated heart. *Acta Anaesthesiologica Scandinavica*, 1978: 22: 649-657.
7. Schuttler J, et al: Infusion strategies to investigate the pharmacokineytics and pharmacodynamics of hypnotic drugs: etomidate as an example. *European Journal of Anaesthesiology*, 1985: 2: 133-142.
8. Goodchild CS, Serrao JM: Cardiovascular effects of propofol in the anaesthetized dog. *British Journal of Anaesthesia*, 1989: 63: 87-92.
9. Major E, et al: Influence of sample site on blood concentrations of ICI 35868. *British Journal of Anaesthesia*, 1983: 55: 371-375.
10. Barratt RL, et al: Kinetics of thiopentone in relation to the site of sampling. *British Journal of Anaesthesia*, 1984: 56: 1385-1391.
11. Reves JG, et al: Negative inotropic effects of midazolam. *Anesthesiology*, 1984: 60: 517.
12. Taeger K, et al: Pulmonary kinetics of fentanyl and alfentanil in surgical patients. *British Journal of Anaesthesia*, 1988: 61: 425-434.
13. Dundee JW, et al: Some factors influencing plasma thiopentone concentrations at awakening. *British Journal of Anaesthesia*, 1980: 52: 101P.
14. Christensen JH, et al: Pharmacokinetics and pharmacodynamics of thiopentone. A comparison between young and elderly patients. *Anaesthesia*, 1982: 37: 398-404.
15. Price HL, et al: Rates of uptake and release of thiopental by human brain; relation to kinetics of thiopental anesthesia. *Anesthesiology*, 1957: 18: 171.
16. Price HL, et al: The uptake of thiopental by body tissues and its relation to the duration of narcosis. *Clinical Pharmacology & Therapeutics*, 1960: 1: 16-22.
17. Kay B: A dose-response relationship for etomidate with some observations on cumulation. *British Journal of Anaesthesia*, 1976: 48: 213-215.
18. Gourlay GK, et al: A double-blind comparison of the efficacy of methadone and morphine in postoperative pain control. *Anesthesiology*, 1986: 64: 322-327.
19. Gourlay GK, et al: Postoperative pain control with methadone: Influence of supplementary methadone doses and blood concentration-response relationships. *Anesthesiology*, 1984: 61: 19-26.
20. Lemmens HJM, et al: Age has no effect on the pharmacodynamics of alfentanil. *Anesthesia and Analgesia*, 1988: 67: 956-960.
21. Aussems ME, Hug CC: Plasma concentrations of alfentanil required to supplement nitrous oxide analgesia for lower abdominal surgery. *British Journal of Anaesthesia*, 1983: 55: supplement 2: 191s-197s.

Chapter 6

Intravenous Infusions

Intravenous infusions are being used with increasing frequency in modern medicine. There are a variety of reasons for this.

- Administration of drugs by intravenous infusion enables a constant plasma drug concentration to be maintained. This is especially important with drugs whose therapeutic concentration range is narrow. The plasma concentrations of such drugs when administered as intermittent intravenous boluses are frequently in the toxic range, or too low to be therapeutic. An example of such a drug is theophylline. Theophylline has a minimum therapeutic plasma concentration of 10 mg/L and a minimum toxic plasma concentration of 20 mg/L [5].

- The dose per unit time of a drug administered by continuous intravenous infusion is lower than if the same drug had been administered intermittently. An example of this is provided by the total dose of midazolam required to maintain hypnosis for a given time. The total dose required to maintain hypnosis is lower when midazolam is administered by constant intravenous infusion, than when administered as intermittent intravenous bolus doses [1].

- Accurate electronically controlled intravenous infusion pumps are becoming increasingly more available in most modern hospitals. These make the administration of drugs by intravenous infusion much easier.

This chapter sets out to explain the methods of administration and the calculations necessary to administer intravenous drug infusions.

CALCULATION OF INFUSION RATE

Once an intravenous drug infusion is started, drug is distributed throughout the V_1 and V_2, as well as being eliminated from the body. Eventually drug concentration in V_2 equals that in V_1, and at this point the rate of drug elimination equals the rate of drug administration. This condition is called **steady state**. Under such circumstances the blood concentration of the drug is constant.

The rate at which a drug is eliminated from the body is only determined by the whole body drug clearance. So calculation of the infusion rate needed to maintain a constant blood or plasma concentration of any drug only requires knowledge of the clearance of that drug. Calculation of the drug infusion rate is therefore **TOTALLY INDEPENDENT** of the number of compartments used in the model describing the kinetic behavior of the drug. The formula used to calculate the steady state drug infusion rate is equation 6.1.

$$Q = C_{ss} \times Cl \qquad (6.1)$$

Q is the drug infusion rate.
C_{ss} is the desired steady state plasma drug concentration.

EXAMPLE 6.1:

A midazolam infusion is used to provide hypnosis/sedation in a 70 kg patient being mechanically ventilated in an intensive care unit. Calculate the infusion rate required.

-   Clearance of Midazolam = Cl = 0.48 L/kg/h [Appendix-A].
-   Midazolam MEC for hypnosis = 0.2 mg/L [Appendix-A].
-   C_{ss} required to be nearly certain that hypnosis will occur = 2 x MEC = 2 x 0.2 = 0.4 mg/L [see chapter 4].
-   Q = C_{ss} x Cl = 0.4 x 0.48 = 0.19 mg/kg/h.
-   For our 70 kg patient this means Q = 70 x 0.192 = 13.4 mg/h.

Equation 5.1 does give the steady state infusion rate required to maintain a set plasma concentration of any given drug. However it says nothing about the speed with which this plasma concentration is achieved after starting an intravenous infusion. The latter can only be calculated with equations 6.2, 6.3, and 6.4.

Concentration-time relationship

The change of drug concentration with time after commencing a constant intravenous infusion of a drug is given by the somewhat daunting series of equations 6.2, 6.3, and 6.4. [see reference 2, page 90, equation 2-172].

$$F = \frac{(k_{el} - \beta)}{(\alpha - \beta)} \qquad (6.2)$$

$$G = \frac{(\alpha - k_{el})}{(\alpha - \beta)} \qquad (6.3)$$

$$C_p = \frac{Q}{Cl} (1 - Fe^{-\alpha t} - Ge^{-\beta t}) \quad (6.4)$$

F and **G** are parameters used in equation 6.4 which are calculated with equations 6.2 and 6.3.
C_p is the blood or plasma drug concentration.
t is time.

If the elapsed time is longer than a time = 4 x $t_{1/2\alpha}$, the term **Fe$^{-\alpha t}$** becomes insignificant and equation 6.4 behaves as a monoexponential equation, [equation 6.5].

$$C_p = \frac{Q}{Cl} (1 - Ge^{-\beta t}) = C_{ss}(1 - Ge^{-\beta t}) \quad (6.5)$$

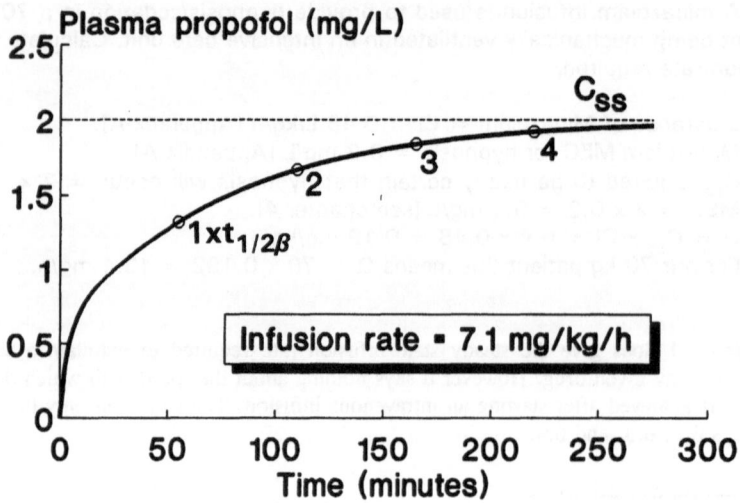

Figure 6.1: Equation 6.4 has been used to show the relationship of the plasma concentration of propofol to multiples of the $t_{1/2\beta}$ for the situation where the drug is infused at a constant rate sufficient to maintain a steady state plasma concentration of 2 mg/L. It takes a time equal to 4 x $t_{1/2\beta}$ to achieve a plasma drug concentration which is slightly higher than 90% of the desired C_{ss}. For propofol, whose $t_{1/2\beta}$ = 55 minutes, the C_{ss} will therefore only be achieved after 4 x 55 = 220 minutes = 3 hours and 40 minutes.

Time required to achieve steady state

Equation 6.5 shows that the time taken for the plasma or blood concentration of a drug administered by constant intravenous infusion to reach the calculated C_{ss} for that infusion rate is mainly determined by the $t_{1/2\beta}$ of that drug. As equation 6.5 is a mono-exponential equation describing a growth process, this means that it will take a time equivalent to 4 x $t_{1/2\beta}$ before the plasma drug concentration is slightly more than 90% of the C_{ss} [see table 1.1 or 3.1]. Figure 6.1 shows this for a constant rate midazolam infusion.

A problem

It takes about 4 x $t_{1/2\beta}$ to achieve a nearly steady state plasma drug concentration after starting a constant intravenous infusion. Steady state is quickly achieved if a drug has a short $t_{1/2\beta}$. However, the period required for the plasma drug concentration to increase to the C_{ss} can be quite long for drugs with a long $t_{1/2\beta}$. This may be quite unacceptable for infusions of some drugs, e.g. infusions of muscle relaxants, hypnotics, inotropic drugs, etc.

EXAMPLE 6.2:

Consider an anxious patient who is administered a constant rate propofol infusion at a rate just sufficient to induce sedation/hypnosis during a surgical procedure performed under regional anesthesia. The desired C_{ss} is equal to the MEC. How long will it take before the desired level of hypnosis or sedation is induced after starting the infusion?

- Propofol MEC for hypnosis = 1 mg/L.
- Desired C_{ss} = MEC = 1 mg/L.
- Propofol $t_{1/2\beta}$ = 55 minutes.
- Time to achieve a plasma midazolam concentration which is ≥ 90% of C_{ss} = 4 x $t_{1/2\beta}$ = 4 x 55 = 220 minutes = 3.67 hours.
- It will take about 3.67 hours for the patient to fall asleep. The operation would have to be delayed for this time, or would have been performed long before hypnosis occurred. Such a dosage regimen is therefore quite impractical.

This is a real problem in clinical practice. Fortunately it can be resolved by administration of a "loading dose".

LOADING DOSE PLUS INFUSION

Consider the situation where a drug is infused into a person in whom none of that drug is present. When the infusion is started, the infused drug is removed from the blood by distribution throughout all the kinetic compartments, as well as by elimination from the body. Once the drug concentration within the pharmacokinetic compartments is the same as in the blood, drug is only lost from the blood by elimination from the body. It takes time to achieve such a steady state situation. This time may be shortened considerably by administering an extra dose of the drug when the drug infusion is started. The purpose of this extra dose is to provide a sufficient amount of drug so that the process of drug distribution will elevate one or more kinetic compartment drug concentrations to a level above or equal to the C_{ss}. Such a dose is called a **loading dose**.

Various methods exist to calculate the magnitude and method of administration of a loading dose. It is these differences between the methods of administration of the loading dose that distinguishes various infusion systems. However, despite the different methods used to calculate a loading dose, the steady state infusion rate is **ALWAYS** calculated with equation 6.1.

Boyes method

If a drug is administered as an intravenous bolus it is first distributed throughout the central compartment. A drug dose required to provide a plasma drug concentration equal to the C_{ss} if the dose were **ONLY** to be distributed throughout the **central compartment** is given by equation 6.6 [3].

$$D_L = C_{ss} \times V_c \qquad (6.6)$$

D_L is the loading dose.

The loading dose is administered at the same time as the infusion is started. Administration of such a loading dose will elevate the plasma concentration to a level no higher than the desired C_{ss}. However, because of rapid redistribution of the injected bolus dose, plus infused drug, from the central compartment to the whole of the distribution volume, the plasma drug concentration rapidly falls below the C_{ss}. Plasma drug concentration then remains below the desired C_{ss} until the infusion eventually elevates the plasma concentration to the C_{ss} after a time equal to $4 \times t_{1/2\beta}$.

One advantage of this type of loading dose is that the plasma drug concentration never rises higher than the desired concentration, and so the chance of toxic or undesired effects is minimized.

EXAMPLE 6.3:

Consider a person to whom an infusion of propofol is administered. The infusion rate is calculated to provide a C_{ss} sufficient to induce hypnosis, and so is 2 x MEC. Use the Boyes method to calculate the loading dose, and also calculate the steady state infusion rate.

- Propofol MEC for hypnosis = 1 mg/L.
- Therefore the desired C_{ss} = 2 x MEC = 2 x 1 = 2 mg/L.
- Propofol V_c = 0.63 L/kg.
- Propofol clearance = 3.55 L/kg/h.

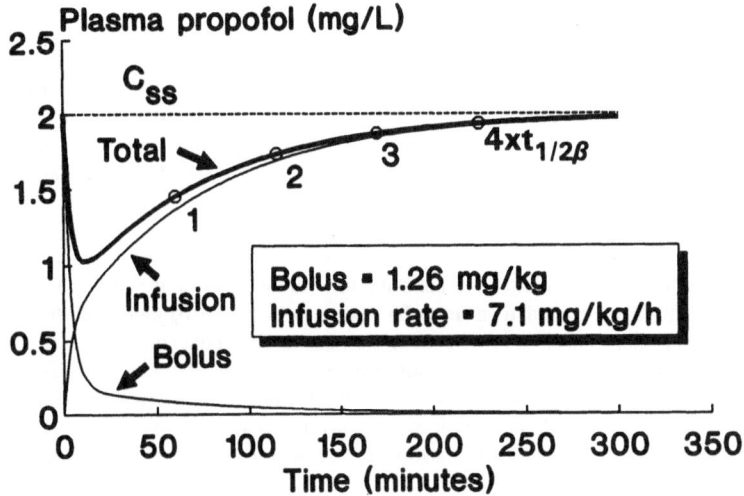

Figure 6.2: A propofol infusion is administered at a rate sufficient to maintain a C_{ss} of 2 mg/L. A loading dose calculated using Boyes' method has been administered when the infusion was started. The total plasma propofol concentration is the sum of the plasma concentrations resulting from the loading bolus dose and the infusion. This figure shows that the plasma propofol concentration falls below the C_{ss} shortly after the loading dose is administered. Plasma propofol concentration will only equal the C_{ss} again after a time equal to 4 x $t_{1/2\beta}$ has passed.

Steady state infusion rate

$Q = C_{ss} \times Cl = 2 \times 3.55 = 7.1$ mg/kg/h.

Loading dose

$D_L = C_{ss} \times V_c = 2 \times 0.63 = 1.26$ mg/kg.

Peak plasma propofol concentration

- Such a loading dose is sufficient to provide an initial plasma propofol concentration of 2 mg/L. This may be confirmed using equation 3.20 or 3.42.
- $C_0 = Dose(A_x + B_x) = 1.26 \times (1.44 + 0.15) = 2$ mg/L.

Redistribution of the bolus dose after administration will cause the plasma propofol concentration to fall below the C_{ss} until about 4 elimination half lives have passed. This has been simulated in figure 6.2.

Mitenko & Ogilvie method

The Boyes loading dose method always carries the penalty of plasma drug concentrations which are lower than the desired C_{ss} for a time equal to 4 x $t_{1/2\beta}$. This is undesirable in many clinical situations. A loading dose calculated with the method of Mitenko and Ogilvie avoids this problem [3,4]. The loading dose is large enough, so that complete distribution of the loading dose throughout the distribution volume will result in a plasma drug concentration equal to the C_{ss}.

$$D_L = C_{ss} \times V_\beta \qquad (6.7)$$

This loading dose is administered at the same time as the infusion is started. The plasma drug concentration is initially elevated to a level far above the C_{ss}. Distribution of the loading dose throughout the drug distribution volume causes the plasma drug concentration to rapidly decline. Plasma drug concentration falls to the C_{ss}, but never drops below this level, [see figure 6.3].

Such a loading dose has the major advantage that the plasma concentration never falls below the desired C_{ss}. However such a loading dose is relatively large. So if the C_{ss} is very close to the toxic concentration, toxic effects may be observed after administration of such a loading dose. An example of such a drug is theophylline.

EXAMPLE 6.4:

Consider an infusion of theophylline for treatment of bronchospasm in an asthmatic patient. Calculate the loading dose using the Mitenko & Ogilvie method, and also calculate the steady state infusion rate required.

- MEC of theophylline for effective bronchodilation = 10 mg/L [5].
- Minimum or THRESHOLD plasma theophylline concentration at which toxic effects occur = 20 mg/L [5].
- So let the desired C_{ss} = 12.5 mg/L.
- $t_{1/2\alpha}$ = 6.5 min: $t_{1/2\beta}$ = 264 min: V_c = 0.15 L/kg : V_β = 0.43 L/kg : Cl = 0.07 L/kg/h [4]. So A_x = 4.58 kg/L: B_x = 2.15 kg/L.

Steady state infusion rate

- $Q = C_{ss} \times Cl$ = 12.5 x 0.07 = 0.88 mg/kg/hour.
- This is equivalent to a dose of 5.3 mg/kg/6 hours.

Loading dose

$D_L = C_{ss} \times V_\beta$ = 12.5 x 0.43 = 5.37 mg/kg.

Peak plasma theophylline concentration

- The initial plasma theophylline concentration achieved with such a loading dose may be calculated using equation 3.20 or 3.42.

-    C_0 = Dose$(A_x + B_x)$ = 5.37(4.58 + 2.15) = 36.11 mg/L. This is higher than the minimum threshold toxic plasma theophylline concentration of 20 mg/L.

Rapid intravenous administration of such a loading dose of theophylline is frequently associated with toxic effects. This example has been simulated in figure 6.3.

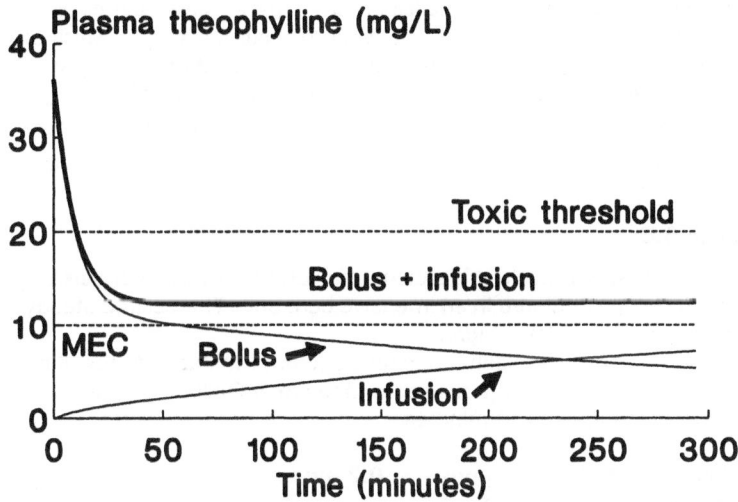

Figure 6.3: This figure shows the plasma theophylline concentration-time curve resulting from an infusion plus loading dose calculated using the method of Mitenko & Ogilvie. Plasma theophylline concentration is the sum of the plasma concentration of theophylline due to the loading dose and the intravenous infusion. The advantages of this techniques are that plasma drug concentration does not fall below the C_{ss} at any time. In addition to this, C_{ss} is achieved in a time slightly longer than 4 x $t_{1/2\alpha}$, which is very much shorter than 4 x $t_{1/2\beta}$.

From the preceding discussion it is evident that the Mitenko and Ogilvie loading dose is one which is clinically very effective. However, with some drugs, there is the problem of potentially high and toxic plasma drug concentrations resulting from such a loading dose, [see example 6.4]. This problem may be solved by administering the loading dose over a time that is long in relation to the $t_{1/2\alpha}$. Significant redistribution of the drug from the central to the peripheral compartments will then occur while the loading dose is being administered. Plasma drug concentration will then not rise to the same levels as when the loading dose is administered much more rapidly. The loading dose may be given by administering it as an infusion or divided into small doses.

Rapid drug infusion

It is evident from the preceding discussion that a loading dose calculated according to the Boyes method is clinically not very useful, while a loading dose calculated according to the method of Mitenko and Ogilvie is clinically very usable, but regrettably may result in undesirably high plasma drug concentrations. There is another way to administer a Mitenko and Ogilvie loading dose. A rapid infusion of a drug at a rate faster than that required to maintain the desired C_{ss} may be used. This is less likely to result in undesirably high plasma drug concentrations.

A simple rule for calculating the duration of such a loading dose infusion is to administer a Mitenko and Ogilvie loading dose over a time equal to about 2-4 x $t_{1/2\alpha}$. Much of the infused loading dose will be (re)distributed by the time the loading dose infusion is stopped. This method does however make the assumption that only an insignificant amount of the drug is eliminated during the loading dose infusion, an assumption which is only a reasonable for drugs with a long elimination half life.

EXAMPLE 6.5:

It is proposed to use a midazolam infusion to provide hypnosis/sedation in a patient being ventilated in an intensive care unit. The desired steady state infusion rate = C_{ss} = 0.2 mg/L.

Calculate the peak plasma concentrations of midazolam resulting from administration of the loading dose as a Mitenko & Ogilvie intravenous bolus, or as an infusion lasting 30 minutes.

- Midazolam MEC for hypnosis = 0.2 mg/L.
- Desired C_{ss} = 0.2 mg/L.
- Midazolam Cl = 0.48 L/kg/h: V_β = 1.9 L/kg: $t_{1/2\alpha}$ = 18.6 min: α = 0.0373: $t_{1/2\beta}$ = 164 min: β = 0.0042: k_{el} = 0.0138: A_x = 1.35: B_x = 0.38.

Mitenko & Ogilvie loading dose

- $D_L = C_{ss} \times V_\beta = 0.2 \times 1.9 = 0.38$ mg/kg.
- Peak plasma concentration resulting from such a loading dose is given by equation 3.20 $C_0 = Dose(A_x + B_x) = 0.38(1.35 + 0.38) = 0.66$ mg/L.

Peak plasma drug concentration resulting from loading infusion

- If the Mitenko and Ogilvie loading dose is administered over 30 minutes as a intravenous infusion, then the possibility of significant drug elimination during the period that the loading dose is administered must be considered. Now 30 minutes is short in relation to the elimination half life of midazolam. This means that little of the loading dose will be

eliminated in this time. Accordingly the total loading dose is NEARLY EQUAL to the Mitenko & Ogilvie loading dose. This means that as 30 minutes = 0.5 hr, that the 0.38 mg/kg Mitenko & Ogilvie loading dose is administered at a rate of rate = 0.38/2 = 0.76 mg/kg/h for 30 minutes.
-   Use equation 6.4 to calculate that the peak plasma midazolam concentration resulting from an infusion of midazolam lasting 30 minutes at a rate of 0.76 mg/kg/h = 0.44 mg/L.

It is evident from this example that the initial plasma midazolam concentration achieved by administering a Mitenko and Ogilvie loading dose by intravenous infusion is significantly less than that due to a bolus dose. The same principle applies to other drugs too.

Example 6.5 shows the advantage of such a loading dose technique. Such a method of administering a Mitenko and Ogilvie loading dose is very appropriate for use with drugs whose therapeutic concentration range is close to their toxic concentration range.

Wagner double infusion method

The rapid initial infusion technique has also been developed in a more formal manner by Wagner (1974) [6]. The drug is also infused rapidly in the first few minutes of the infusion. Subsequently the infusion rate is slowed down to the rate required to maintain the C_{ss}. Both the rate and duration of the first infusion are calculated so the plasma concentration of the drug never falls below the C_{ss} once the infusion rate is reduced to that required to maintain the steady state plasma drug concentration. The total dose of drug infused during the initial rapid infusion is the same as a bolus dose calculated according to the method of Mitenko & Ogilvie.

Rate and duration of the first infusion are based on the rate of the second infusion according to equation 6.8.

$$Q_1 = \frac{Q_2}{(1 - e^{-\beta T})} \tag{6.8}$$

Q_1 is the rate of the initial loading dose infusion.
Q_2 is the rate of second steady state infusion.
T is the desired duration of initial loading dose infusion.

If time to onset of drug effect is to be short, then T must also be short. This nearly always means that T is also very short in relation to the $t_{1/2\beta}$ of the drug used too. Under such circumstances very little drug is eliminated during the time the loading dose is administered. So equation 6.8 may be usefully approximated by equation 6.9 which is simpler to use in a clinical setting.

$$Q_1 = \frac{Q_2}{\beta T} \qquad (6.9)$$

However, while equation 6.9 can be used to calculate a loading dose infusion, it says nothing about the peak plasma drug concentration achieved when such a loading dose is administered. Equation 6.4 must be used to calculate the peak plasma concentration achieved by such an infusion.

EXAMPLE 6.6:

An asthmatic patient is to be administered a theophylline infusion. The patient has a history of intermittent tachyarrhythmias, so the physician does not wish the plasma theophylline concentration to exceed the lower toxic threshold concentration. Calculate the Mitenko & Ogilvie loading dose, the initial infusion rate using the Wagner double infusion technique, and the peak plasma concentrations arising from these loading doses. Also calculate the steady state infusion rate.

- Theophylline MEC = 10 mg/L [5].
- Minimum threshold plasma theophylline concentration for toxic effects = 20 mg/L [5].
- Theophylline kinetics [4]: $t_{1/2\alpha}$ = 6.5 minutes : $t_{1/2\beta}$ = 264 minutes : α = 0.106 min^{-1}: β = 0.002622 min^{-1}: V_c = 0.15 L/kg: V_β = 0.43 L/kg: Cl = 0.00116 L/kg/min = 0.07 L/kg/h: A_x = 4.58 kg/L : B_x = 2.15 kg/L : k_{el} = 0.0078 min^{-1}.

C_{ss} and duration of initial infusion

- Let the initial infusion in the Wagner double infusion technique last 30 minutes. This is long in relation to the $t_{1/2\alpha}$, allowing time for distribution of the infused drug. It is also short in relation to the $t_{1/2\beta}$, and so very little drug will be eliminated during the loading infusion.
- Let the desired C_{ss} = 12.5 mg/L, a concentration well within the therapeutic range.

Steady state infusion rate

$Q_2 = C_{ss} \times Cl = 12.5 \times 0.00116 = 0.0145$ mg/kg/min.

Wagner initial infusion rate and peak concentration

- The initial loading infusion rate = Q_1 = $Q_2/\beta T$ = 0.0145/(0.002622 × 30) = 0.1843 mg/kg/min.
- The total dose of theophylline administered during 30 minutes of Q_1 = 30 × 0.1843 = 5.53 mg/kg.

- Peak plasma concentration achieved with the initial infusion is given by equation 6.4 = C_p = 19.03 mg/L.

Mitenko & Ogilvie loading dose and peak concentration

- Mitenko & Ogilvie loading dose = D_L = C_{ss} x V_β = 12.5 x 0.43 = 5.37 mg/kg.
- Peak plasma theophylline concentration due to Mitenko & Ogilvie loading dose = C = Dose(A_x + B_x) = 5.37(4.58 + 2.15) = 36.14 mg/L.

Here again the double infusion technique is superior to a Mitenko & Ogilvie loading dose. The Wagner double infusion system is less likely to cause toxic plasma theophylline concentrations.

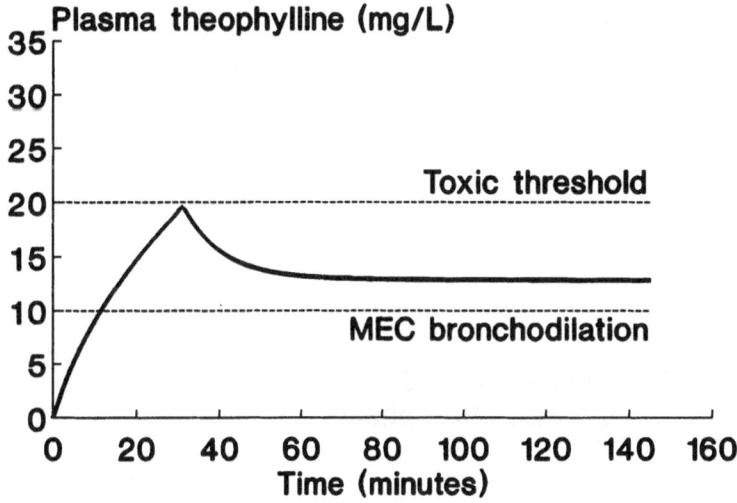

Figure 6.4: This figure shows the change of plasma theophylline concentration with time when it is administered according to the double infusion technique of Wagner [6]. The kinetic data used are from Mitenko & Ogilvie [4], the desired C_{ss} is 12.5 mg/L, and the initial infusion is administered over 30 minutes.

BET infusion technique

BET stands for Bolus-Elimination-Transfer, which is the name of an intravenous bolus loading dose and infusion system. This technique is capable of instantly providing, and maintaining a plasma drug concentration at a level equal to that required [1]. The difference between this bolus-infusion technique and others is the variable drug infusion rate.

1.   The bolus loading dose is calculated according to the method of Boyes [see equation 6.6]. This immediately elevates the plasma drug concentration to the C_{ss}.

2.   Simultaneously with the administration of the bolus dose, an infusion of the same drug is started. The infusion rate is initially very high. This maintains the plasma drug concentration at the C_{ss} while drug is distributed throughout the V_β. As the drug concentration in V_2 approaches that in V_1, the rate of drug loss from V_1 decreases, and the infusion rate is decreased. Finally, when drug concentration in V_2 equals the drug concentration in V_1, drug is only lost by elimination.

Equation 6.10 describes the change of infusion rate with time when the BET intravenous infusion technique is used.

$$Q = V_1 \cdot C_{ss}(k_{el} + k_{12} \cdot e^{-t \cdot k21}) \tag{6.10}$$

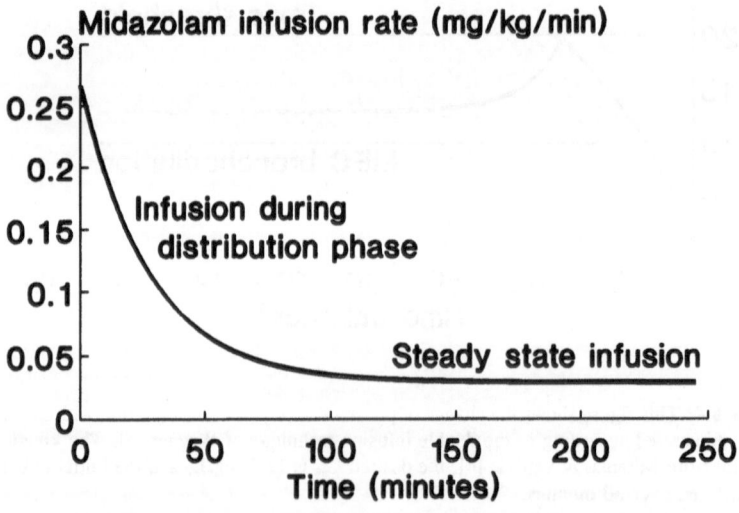

Figure 6.5: This figure shows the change of infusion rate with time for a midazolam infusion administered using the BET drug administration scheme. The infusion is calculated to provide a midazolam C_{ss} = 0.4 mg/L.

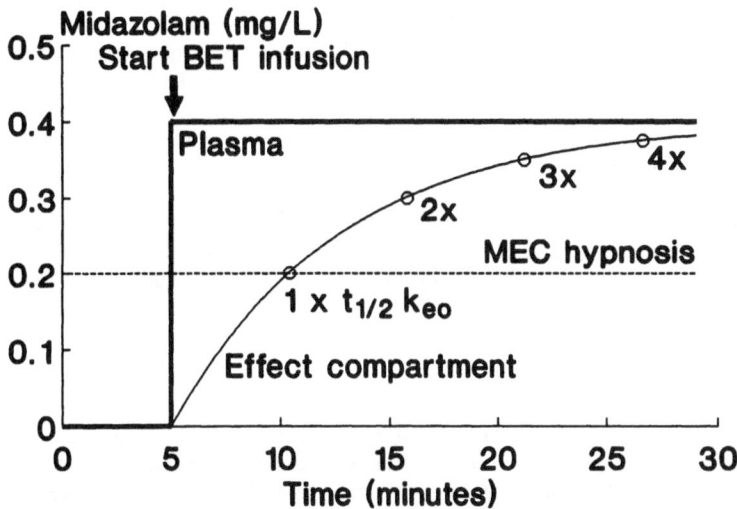

Figure 6.6: Plasma and effect compartment midazolam concentrations resulting from a BET infusion which is used to maintain a plasma midazolam concentration of 0.4 mg/L. This figure shows that the plasma midazolam concentration is instantly elevated and maintained at the C_{ss}. The speed with which the effect compartment concentration becomes equal to that in plasma is then only determined by two factors. One, the difference between the C_{ss} and the MEC for midazolam. In this case the MEC is for hypnosis. Two, the $t_{1/2}k_{eo}$ of midazolam. Note the similarity between this figure and figures 4.9 and 4.12.

The necessity for a programmable mechanical or computer controlled infusion pump is evident when equation 6.10 and figure 6.5 are studied. This is unfortunate, as such pumps are neither cheap nor readily available. So this otherwise theoretically ideal technique is doomed to be used in only a few wealthy or fortunate clinics.

Practical common-sense method

The above methods for calculating and providing a loading dose are all very well, but clinical practice is sometimes quite different. There are a variety of reasons for this.

- Minimal to no equipment to administer intravenous drug infusions is available. Perhaps all that is available is an intravenous infusion and a watch with a second hand to count the drip rate.

- Some patients may be hemodynamically unstable. The causes of this range from hypovolemia, other drugs, or myocardial depression, to autonomic neuropathy. If drugs which cause cardiovascular depression are administered to such persons, profound cardiovascular depression may occur. Such cardiovascular depression may be severe enough to induce myocardial ischemia or infarction in some patients. In patients with elevated cerebral pressure, a reduction of arterial blood pressure may cause a lethal period of cerebral ischemia. In such situations it is better not to administer a Mitenko & Ogilvie loading dose of any drug which may cause cardiovascular depression.

- Some patients receive infusions of cardioactive drugs. A loading dose of such a cardioactive drug may cause a greater effect than what is desired. Here too, it is not advisable to administer a Mitenko & Ogilvie loading dose of the drug to be infused.

EXAMPLE 6.7:

Consider a patient who has sustained severe cerebral trauma together with multiple long bone fractures. This has caused markedly elevated intracranial pressure together with hypovolemia. To make matters even worse, the patient is hypoxic due to fat emboli from his multiple fractures. The patient is contusional and extremely irritable due to both the head injury as well as hypoxia. It is decided to mechanically hyperventilate the patient using a midazolam infusion to sedate the patient and to reduce restlessness.

Calculate the steady state infusion rate and the Mitenko and Ogilvie loading dose. Estimate the chances of developing myocardial depression from the loading dose.

Parameters

- Midazolam MEC for hypnosis = 0.2 mg/L [see appendix-A].
- Midazolam MEC for myocardial depression = 15 mg/L [see table 5.1 in chapter 5].
- Midazolam kinetic parameters: V_β = 1.91 L/kg : Cl = 0.48 L/kg/h : A_x = 1.35 kg/L: B_x = 0.38 kg/L.

Desired C_{ss}

The desired C_{ss} which will almost certainly guarantee that the patient will sleep or be heavily sedated without developing hypotension due to myocardial depression = C_{ss} = 2 x MEC = 2 x 0.2 = 0.4 mg/L, [see chapter 4].

Steady state infusion rate

Steady state infusion rate = Q = C_{ss} x Cl = 0.4 x 0.48 = 0.192 mg/kg/h = 13.44 mg/70 kg/h.

Mitenko & Ogilvie loading dose

It is desired to administer a loading dose at the start of the infusion. A loading dose calculated according to the method of Mitenko & Ogilvie.

$$D_L = C_{ss} \times V_\beta = 0.4 \times 1.91 = 0.764 \text{ mg/kg} = 53.48 \text{ mg/70 kg}$$

Peak plasma midazolam concentration

The peak plasma midazolam concentration due to such a loading dose can be calculated using equations 3.20 or 3.42.

$$C_0 = \text{Dose}(A_x + B_x) = 0.764(1.35 + 0.35) = 1.3 \text{ mg/L}$$

This is lower than the MEC for myocardial depression for midazolam of 15 mg/L shown in table 5.1. However, such a dose (53.48 mg) of midazolam is certainly associated with myocardial depression. This is presumably due to pre-recirculation phase midazolam concentrations which are much higher than the peak concentration calculated here.

The effect of such a large loading dose of midazolam would be to cause profound cardiovascular depression. This may reduce the cerebral perfusion pressure so much that the patient would become decerebrate. In such a situation it is always better to start the infusion without any loading dose. Then intermittently administer doses of 2.5-5 mg midazolam/70 kg according to the degree of restlessness. Provided that the hemodynamic condition of the patient permits, these small intermittent boluses are continued until the patient no longer requires extra sedation. Such a technique makes it possible to administer a loading dose safely under these difficult circumstances. In fact this technique is widely applied in practice for just this reason.

The method described in example 6.7 is often applied in clinical anesthetic practice. An infusion of a drug is administered at a predetermined rate. Small intravenous boluses of the same drug are intermittently administered, or the infusion rate is occasionally increased, until the desired effect is maintained by the infusion alone. This method guarantees that no excessively large doses of the drug are suddenly administered. Such a method of drug administration is readily applicable to infusions of vasodilators, vasoconstrictors, inotropics, hypnotics, sedatives, opiates, muscle relaxants as the therapeutic or physiological effects achieved with these drugs are readily assessed or measured.

INCREASING THE INFUSION RATE

Sometimes the effect of an intravenous infusion is less than that which is desired. So the infusion rate must be increased. However, after increasing the infusion rate to a new level, it will take a time $= 4 \times t_{1/2\beta}$ before the new desired C_{ss} is achieved. This will take too much time for most clinical purposes, and so a new supplementary loading dose is required. How can this supplementary loading dose be calculated?

The assumptions and reasoning behind such a calculation are listed below.

1. Assume the initial infusion has reached steady state. This is usually the situation and is accordingly a very reasonable assumption.

2. As the initial infusion has already reached steady state, no loading dose need be administered for an infusion of that drug up to that rate.

3. A loading dose is required to increase the drug concentration in all the kinetic compartments to the new desired C_{ss}. So the loading dose required is one which is appropriate for an infusion rate which is the difference between the initial infusion rate and the new higher infusion rate.

The incremental Mitenko & Ogilvie loading dose is expressed by equation 6.11, which is an extension of equation 6.7.

$$D_L = V_\beta(C_{ss(2)} - C_{ss(1)}) \qquad (6.11)$$

$C_{ss(1)}$ is the initial C_{ss}.
$C_{ss(2)}$ is the new desired C_{ss}.

EXAMPLE 6.8:

Let us consider an unfortunate patient being sedated with a midazolam infusion while undergoing mechanical ventilation in an intensive care unit. The patient is restless despite a midazolam $C_{ss} = 0.2$ mg/L. Accordingly it is decided to increase the midazolam C_{ss} to 0.4 mg/L. Calculate the necessary supplementary loading dose.

-   $C_{ss(1)} = 0.2$ mg/L.
-   $C_{ss(2)} = 0.4$ mg/L.

-   Midazolam $V_\beta = 1.91$ mg/L: Cl $= 0.48$ L/kg/h.

-   Use equation 6.11. The supplementary loading dose required for the increased infusion rate $= D_L = V_\beta(C_{ss(2)} - C_{ss(1)}) = 1.91(0.4 - 0.2) = 0.382$ mg/kg.

This method of calculation is applicable to intravenous infusions of any other drug too.

STOPPING AN INTRAVENOUS INFUSION

An intravenous infusion of a drug is eventually stopped because the drug is no longer required. Unfortunately, a drug is unable to be immediately removed from the body after intravenous administration. Most drugs also cannot be antagonized as can heparin, the opiates or benzodiazepines. So all that can be done is to wait for the plasma drug concentration to fall due to distribution and elimination.

Equations 6.12, 6.13 and 6.14 describe the change of plasma drug concentration with time after terminating any intravenous infusion, [equation 2-195a, page 100, reference 2].

$$X = \frac{(k_{el} - \beta)(1 - e^{-\alpha T})}{(\alpha - \beta)} \qquad (6.12)$$

$$Y = \frac{(k_{el} - \alpha)(1 - e^{-\beta T})}{(\alpha - \beta)} \qquad (6.13)$$

$$C_p = \frac{Q}{Cl}(Xe^{-\alpha(t - T)} - Ye^{-\beta(t - T)}) \qquad (6.14)$$

X and **Y** are parameters used in equation 6.14, and which are calculated with equations 6.12 and 6.13.
T is the duration of the infusion.
t is elapsed time after starting the infusion.

Equation 6.14 is rather large and complex. It is impossible to use it in any other setting other than theoretical, or by clinicians equipped with programmable calculators or computers. It is essentially a bi-exponential decay equation, whose properties are similar to those of the familiar bi-exponential decay equation of the 2-compartment kinetic model.

So regardless of how long an infusion lasts, the processes of both distribution and elimination determine the rate of decline of the plasma drug concentration. The total amount of drug in the body at the termination of an infusion is what determines the duration of drug effect after stopping the infusion. This is simply a question of the total amount, or dose, of drug remaining in the body at the end of the infusion. A nice illustration of this point is given by the duration of effect of propofol after steady state infusions with the same C_{ss} have been administered for different lengths of time [see fig. 6.7].

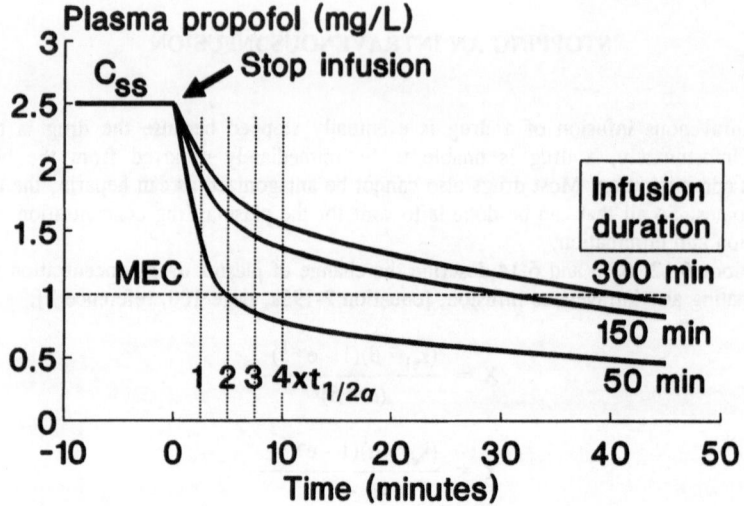

Figure 6.7: A propofol infusion has been administered at a C_{ss} of 2.5 mg/L for periods of 50, 150 and 300 minutes before the infusion was stopped at time = 0 minutes. The time it takes for the plasma propofol concentration to drop below the MEC is determined by the total amount of drug in the body, which is a function of the duration of the infusion, as well as the processes of distribution and elimination.

Unfortunately the duration of the effect can really only be calculated exactly with equation 6.14. However for practical purposes, it may be said the if the infusion was longer than 4 x $t_{1/2\beta}$, then the drug concentration in all kinetic compartments is about the same, and the rate of drug concentration decline is mainly determined by elimination.

EXAMPLE 6.9:

Our hypothetical patient, sedated with midazolam while being mechanically ventilated, has recovered somewhat. The treating physicians wish to allow him to wake up before stopping mechanical ventilation. The midazolam C_{ss} at this time is 0.4 mg/L. Approximately how long will it take this patient to awaken?

- Midazolam MEC for hypnosis = 0.2 mg/L.
- The $t_{1/2\beta}$ of midazolam = 164 minutes = 2.73 hours.

- C_{ss} = 0.4 mg/L at the time the infusion was stopped.

- After a time = 1 x $t_{1/2\beta}$ = 2.73 hours, the plasma midazolam concentration approximately halves from 0.4 mg/L to about 0.2 mg/L. This is equal to the MEC for hypnosis. So the patient will awaken soon after 2.73 hours have elapsed after stopping the infusion.

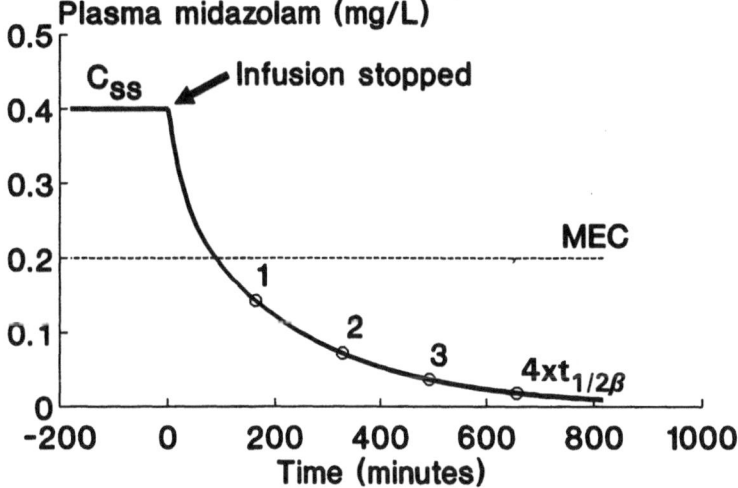

Figure 6.8: This figure shows the exponential decline of the plasma drug concentration after stopping an infusion of midazolam which had continued for longer than 4 x $t_{1/2\beta}$, and so had achieved concentration equilibrium in all kinetic compartments. The rate of decline of plasma drug concentration is determined mainly by the elimination half life.

The method of calculation is the same for any other drug administered by intravenous infusion.

<h2 style="text-align:center">REFERENCES</h2>

1. Lauven PM, et al: Ein pharmakokinetisch begründetes Infusionsmodell für Midazolam. Eine mikroprozessorgesteuerte Applikationsform zur Erreichung konstanter Plasmaspiegel. *Der Anaesthesist*, 1982: 31: 15-20.

2.   Wagner,J.G.,"Fundamentals of Clinical Pharmacokinetics", published Drug Intelligence Publications, INC., Hamilton, Illinois, U.S.A., 1979, ISBN 0-914678-20-4.
3.   Rigg JRA, Wong TY: A method for achieving rapidly steady-state blood concentrations of i.v. drugs. *British Journal of Anaesthesia*, 1981: 53: 1247-1257.
4.   Mitenko PA, Ogilvie RI: Rapidly achieved plasma concentration plateaus, with observations on theophylline kinetics. *Clinical Pharmacology & Therapeutics*, 1972: 13: 329-335.
5.   Hendeles L, Weinberger M: Theophylline. A "state of the art" review. *Pharmacotherapy*, 1983: 3: 2-44.
6.   Wagner JG: A safe method for rapidly achieving plasma concentration plateaus. *Clinical Pharmacology & Therapeutics*, 1974: 16: 691-700.

Chapter 7

Body Weight and Composition

The individuals making up a population vary considerably. Body weight varies with age, and also among individuals of any givien age. The other major difference between individuals in a population is in body composition. A person may be lean, average, muscular or obese.

The purpose of this chapter is to provide a general discussion of the effects of variations of body weight and composition on the kinetics of anesthetic drugs. Subsequent chapters will discuss specific conditions associated with variations of body weight and composition. General principles discussed in this chapter are applied to these problem.

BODY WEIGHT

The volumes throughout which a drug can distribute are large in a large body, and small in a small body. A similar relationship is approximately true for drug clearance too. A larger body has larger kidneys and liver, as well as other organs which eliminate drugs. Accordingly drugs kinetic parameters are usually related to body weight. However this relationship is not as simple as this introductory discussion would seem to imply.

Age related changes in body weight and kinetics

Body weight increases after birth until adulkt weight. During growth the weights of all the organs which metabolize and excrete drugs also increase with age, as do all the tissue volumes throughout which drugs ditribute. So the ABSOLUTE magnitues of kinetic drug volumes, and clearance increase with age until adult weight is achieved. Anexample of this is provided by the changes of morphine distribution volume and clearance with age [figure 7.1].

Not only do the sizes of nearly all organs increase during growth, but their weights in relation to body weight also change. These changes affect drug kinetics by altering the relative composition of the body.

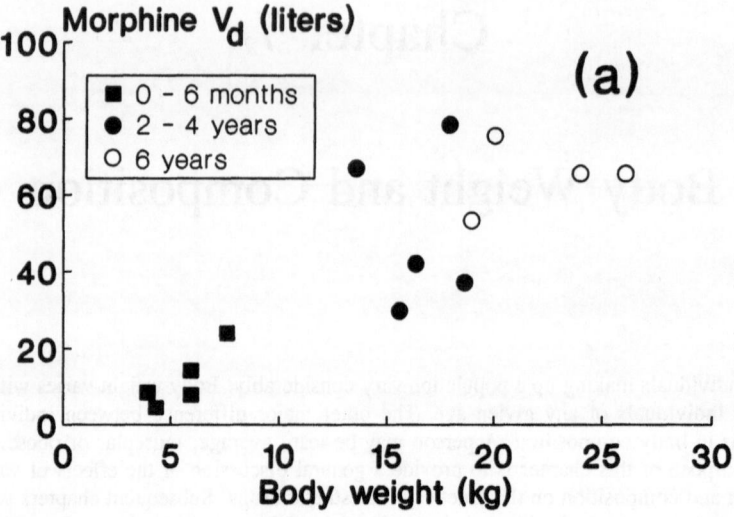

Figure 7.1: Both the total distribution volume [see fig 7.1a] and the clearance [see fig 7.1b] of morphine increase with age in children because body weight and sizes of organs increase with age [1].

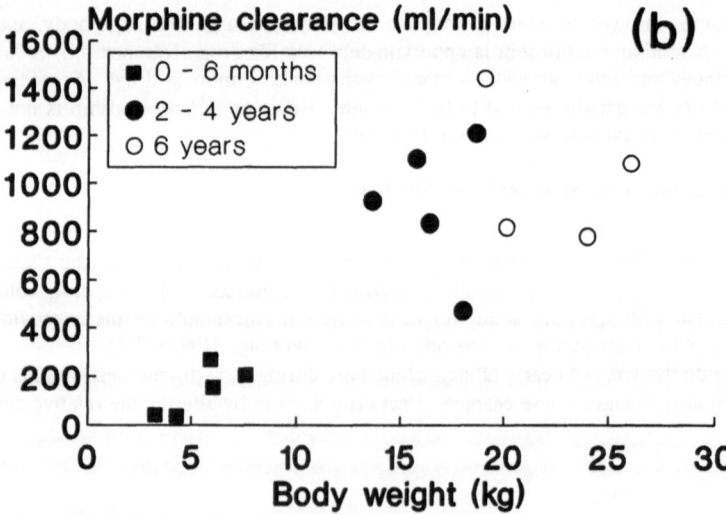

Table 7.1

Correlation coefficients between body weight in ADULTS and total V_c, V_d and Cl for various drugs. A correlation coefficient greater than 0.5 is very significant, while a coefficient less than 0.5 indicates a weak relationship, or that there is none.

	Correlation coefficients for:		
DRUG	V_c	V_d	Cl
Thiopental [2]	0.2	0.18	0.61*
Etomidate [3]	0.67*	0.64*	0.23
Lorazepam [4]	0.12	0.86*	0.48
Alfentanil [5]	0.52*	0.1	0.06
Pancuronium [6]	0.35	0.57*	0.11
Gallamine [7]	0.66*	0.55*	0.77*
Alcuronium [8]	0.14	0.07	0.33

* Means that the correlation of the kinetic parameter with body weight is highly significant.

Relation of kinetic parameters to body weight in adults

Adult body weight varies considerably. Some persons may weigh as much as 200 kg, while others may only weigh as little as 45 kg. The weight of the "average" healthy adult is about 70 kg. However, in practical terms for the purposes of pharmacokinetic studies, adult body weight may be defined as a body weight above 45 kg.

Unfortunately the relation of body weight in adults to the kinetic properties of anesthetic drugs has not been extensively studied. Studies for which data are available show a very inconsistent relation of kinetic parameters with body weight [see table 7.1 and figures 7.2, 7.3, 7.4 and 7.5].KInetic parameters are related to body weight for some drugs, while no such relationship is evident for others. It is also clear from the various figures and tables in this chapter that there is also a wide variation in the magnitude of any one parameter at any particular body weight. There are various reasons for this. Most of the study groups used to determine the kinetics of anesthetic drugs were small, and there were relatively large differences between individuals in each study group. The study groups did not consist of homogneous groups. There were perrsons of different sexes, ages, body build, body composition and with differing coexisting diseases.

Figure 7.2: Relationship of thiopental kinetics to body weight in adults [2].

Figure 7.3: Relationship of alfentanil kinetics to body weight in adults [5].

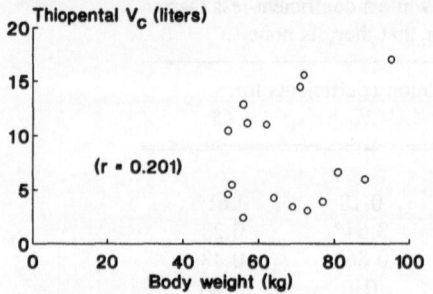

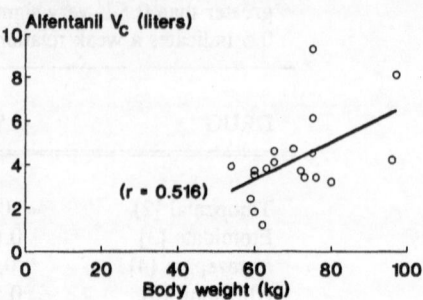

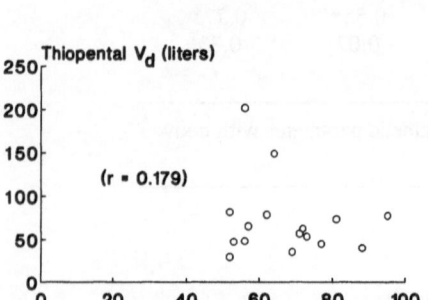

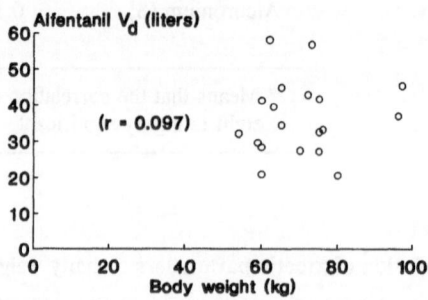

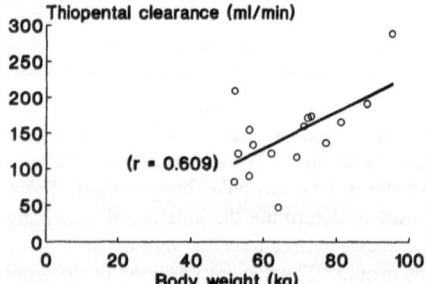

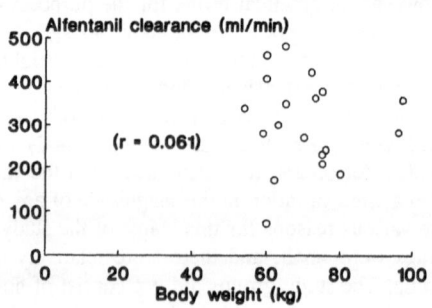

Figure 7.4: Relationship of alcuronium kinetics to body weight in adults [5].

Figure 7.5: Relationship of pancuronium kinetics to body weight in adults [6].

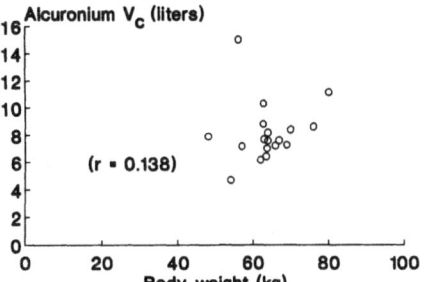

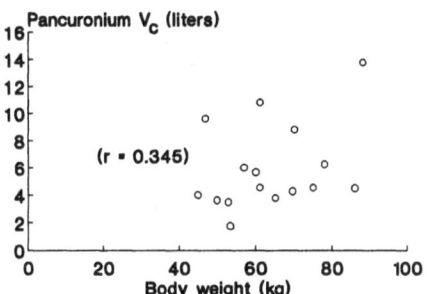

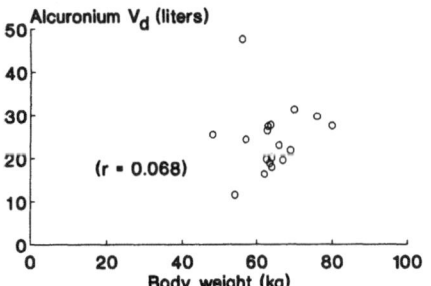

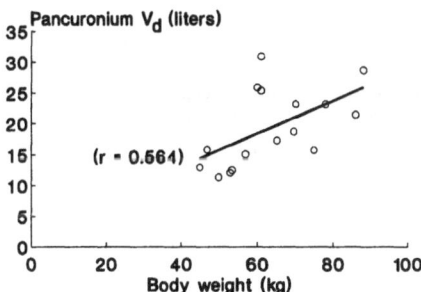

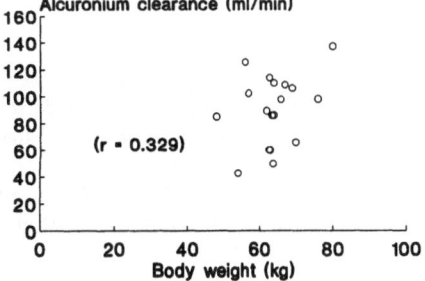

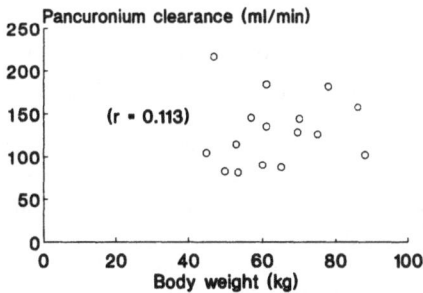

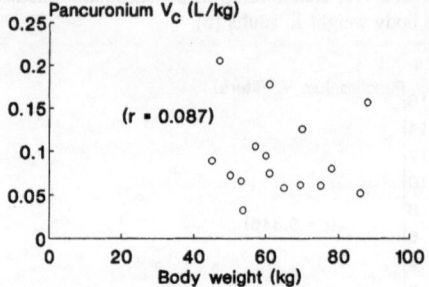

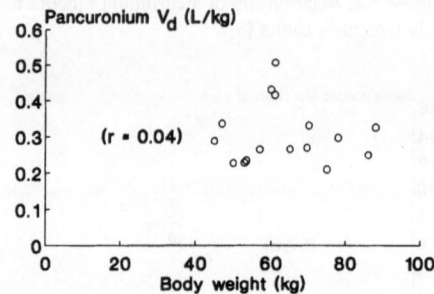

Figure 7.6: Here are the same data for pancuronium kinetics as were presented in figures 7.5a, 7.5b and 7.5c. Only here the kinetic terms have been weight adjusted and accordingly expressed in terms of L/kg and ml/min/kg. This effectively removes any weight dependance of these parameters.

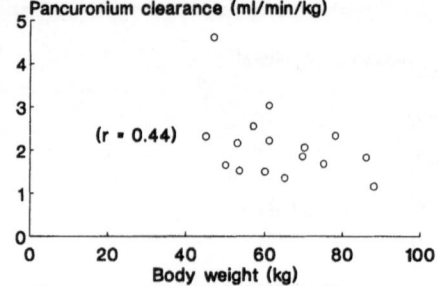

Weight adjusted pharmacokinetic parameters

Weight adjustment is one simple method by which interpersonal variability of pharmacokinetic parameters amy be reduced. This is not a complex method. All that is required is to divide the absolute value of a pharamacokinetic parameter for a given person with the body weight of that person. Kinetic parameters are then expressed in terms of volume/kilogram body weight, e.g. L/kg, ml/kg etc. The same can also be done for clearance, which is then expressed as l/h/kg, or ml/min/kg. Such a procedure then removes any relationship of these parameters to body weight, if any such a relationship ever existed. The accuracy of kinetic parameters of drugs which are not related to body weight are not affected by weight adjustment.

Weight adjustment increases the utility, but not the accuracy, of pharamacokinetic parameters. Kinetic parameters which have been weight adjusted may be applied to adults of all wights. They may even be applied, with reservations, to children too.

BODY COMPOSITION AND KINETIC VOLUMES

Body composition is determined by the relative proportions of bone, skeletal muscle, adipose tissue and extracellular fluid. Bone may be ignored for the purposes of pharmacokinetic analysis of anesthetic drugs. It is a tissue which plays no role in the short or long term distribution and elimination of these drugs. Skeletal muscle, adipose tissue and extracellular fluid account for at least 65% of body weight [see table 2.3, and 7.2]. It is the relative proportions and absolute volumes of these three tissues which are the main determinants of the pharmacokinetic volumes of anesthetic drugs.

Table 7.2
[Data from table 2.3]

TISSUE	Volume of tissue (% body weight)	Interstitial fluid volume of tissue (% tissue weight)
Extracellular fluid	20-26%	100%
Adipose tissue	16-36%	18%
Skeletal muscle	43%	12%

Chapters 2 and 3 have already briefly referred to the influence of body composition on drug kinetic volumes. This discussion will now be extended to more specific examples of how whole body composition affects the kinetics of anesthetic drugs.

Extracellular fluid volume (ECFV)

ECFV is one of the factors determining body composition. Variations of normal physiology as well as pathological conditions can change the ECFV. Conditions causing hypovolemia and dehydration all reduce the ECFV. ECFV is increased above normal adult levels of 20-26% of body weight during pregnancy, in infants under one year of age, and in persons with peripheral edema due to hypoproteinemia, hepatic, renal, endocrine or cardiac diseases.

Change of ECFV is mainly of importance for the kinetics of highly ionized and fat-insoluble drugs. The neuromuscular blocking agents are examples of such drugs. These mainly distribute to the ECFV [9, and appendix-A]. For example, the ECFV expressed as a percentage of body weight is higher in neonates than in adults. This explains the larger distribution volumes of nondepolarizing muscle relaxants in infants and neonates as compared to adults [10,11, and see table 7.3].

Table 7.3.

Effect of differences in ECFV between adults and infants on the weight adjusted V_d of d-tubocurarine [10] and vecuronium [11].

DRUG		ECFV (% body weight)	V_d (L/kg)
d-Tubocurarine	neonates (0-2 months)	39%[12,13]	0.74
	adults (12-30 years)	20-26%[14,15]	0.3
Vecuronium	infants (3-11 months)	28-39%[12,13]	0.36
	adults (29-69 years)	20-26%[14,15]	0.27

The same relationship between distribution volume and ECFV occurs with other depolarizing and non-depolarizing muscle relaxants. This relationship also applies to other fat insoluble drugs. For example, the distribution volume of dobutamine is directly proportional to the degree of peripheral edema in persons with cardiac failure [21].

Total body fat

Two persons with the same body weight may have quite different body compositions. One may be obese while the other may have a normal body composition. The difference between two such persons is the total and relative body fat content. In the average adult, total body fat is about 16-35% of body weight. An obese person has a higher percentage total body fat content. Some morbidly obese persons may have a body fat content which is as much as 60% of the body weight. Such a difference in relative body fat content has a marked effect on the distribution volumes of many drugs. This is especially true for fat soluble drugs.

Fat soluble drugs

The absolute and weight adjusted distribution volumes of fat soluble drugs are increased in persons with a relatively high total body fat content, and vice versa. Consider the drug thiopental. Thiopental is very soluble in adipose tissue, having a fat/plasma partition coefficient of 11 [appendix-B]. So the distribution volume of thiopental is larger in obese persons than in individuals with an average body build [16,17, see also table 7.4].

Table 7.4.

The difference between the weight adjusted V_d of thiopental for obese and non-obese females related to percentage body fat content. (Data for age, height and weight, as well as V_d are mean values from Jung et al (1982) [16]. ECFV and the body fat content were calculated using the equations of Bruce et al 1980) [15].)

BODY BUILD	Age (yrs)	Weight (kg)	Height (cm)	ECFV (% BW)	Body fat (% BW)	V_d (L/kg)
NON-OBESE	34.5	57.4	164	27	24	1.95
OBESE	33	137.9	168	19	45	7.94

BW is an abbreviation for body weight.

Table 7.5.

The weight adjusted V_d of vecuronium in both obese and non-obese persons is compared. (Kinetic data are from Matteo et al (1989) [18]. ECFV was calculated using the formulae of Moore et al (1963) [20].)

BODY BUILD	Age (yrs)	Weight (kg)	ECFV (% BW)	Body fat (% BW)	V_d (L/kg)
NON-OBESE	44.5	62	26.5	17	0.4
OBESE	52.4	94	23	51	0.384

BW is an abbreviation for body weight.

Fat insoluble drugs

The distribution volumes of fat insoluble drugs such as the non-depolarizing muscle relaxants is the ECFV. Percentage interstitial fluid volume in adipose tissue is about the same as in muscle tissue [table 7.2], which means that ECFV expressed as a percentage of body weight is about the same in obese as in non-obese persons. Because of this the weight adjusted V_d of fat insoluble drugs, expressed as L/kg body weight, is about the same in obese and non-obese persons. Indeed this has been confirmed for two non-depolarizing muscle relaxants, vecuronium [18] and metocurine [19].

CONCLUSIONS

There is a relationship between body weight and the kinetic parameters of many drugs used in anesthesia. However, it is a very variable and inconsistent relationship which also depends on other factors such as age and body composition.

Age, body length and weight are easily measured, but body composition is not so easily determined in a quantitative manner in busy clinical practice. This means that all the anesthesiologist can do is make a rough qualitative estimate of body composition, and use this as a guide to adjust dosage and drug administration regimens. In practice this means that weight adjusted kinetic parameters are used to calculate a drug dose which is then increased or decreased according to the body composition and clinical condition of the patient.

REFERENCES

1.   Olkkola KT, et al: Kinetics and dynamics of postoperative intravenous morphine in children. *Clinical Pharmacology & Therapeutics*, 1988: 44: 128-135.
2.   Christensen JH, et al: Pharmacokinetics of thiopentone in a group of young women and a group of young men. *British Journal of Anaesthesia*, 1980: 52: 913-917.
3.   Fragen RJ, et al: A pharmacokinetically designed etomidate infusion regimen for hypnosis. *Anesthesia and Analgesia*, 1983: 62: 654-660.
4.   Greenblatt DJ, et al: Lorazepam kinetics in the elderly. *Clinical Pharmacology & Therapeutics*, 1979: 76: 103-113.
5.   Van Beem H, et al: Pharmacokinetics of alfentanil during and after a fixed rate infusion. *British Journal of Anesthesia*, 1989: 62: 610-615.
6.   Somogyi AA, et al: Combined i.v. bolus and infusion of pancuronium bromide. *British Journal of Anaesthesia*, 1978: 50: 575-581.
7.   Shanks CA, et al: Gallamine administered by combined bolus and infusion. *Anesthesia and Analgesia*, 1982: 61: 847-852.
8.   Walker J, et al: Clinical pharmacokinetics of alcuronium chloride in man. *European Journal of Clinical Pharmacology*, 1980: 17: 449-457.
9.   Cohen EN, et al: The distribution and fate of d-tubocurarine. *Journal of Pharmacology and Experimental Therapeutics*, 1965: 147: 120-129.
10.   Fisher DM, et al: Pharmacokinetics and pharmacodynamics of d-tubocurarine in infants, children, and adults. *Anesthesiology*, 1982: 57: 203-208.
11.   Fisher DM, et al: Vecuronium kinetics and dynamics in anesthetized infants and children. *Clinical Pharmacology & Therapeutics*, 1985: 37: 402-406.
12.   Friis-Hansen B: Body water compartments in children: Changes during growth and related changes in body composition. *Pediatrics*, 1961: 28: 169-181.

13. Friis-Hansen B: Body composition during growth. In vivo measurements and biochemical data correlated to differential anatomical growth. *Pediatrics*, 1971: 47: 264-274.
14. Skrabal F, et al: Equations for the prediction of normal values for exchangeable sodium, exchangeable potassium, extracellular volume, and total body water. *British Medical Journal*, 1973 2: 37-38.
15. Bruce A, et al: Prediction of normal body potassium, body water and body fat in adults on the basis of body height, body weight and age. *Scandinavian Journal of Clinical & Laboratory Investigation*, 1980: 40: 461-463.
16. Jung D, et al: Thiopental disposition in lean and obese patients undergoing surgery. *Anesthesiology*, 1982: 56: 269-274.
17. Mayersonn M, et al: Thiopental kinetics in obese surgical patients. *Anesthesiology*, 1981: 55: A178.
18. Matteo RS, et al: Pharmacokinetics and pharmacodynamics of vecuronium in the obese surgical patient. *Anesthesia and Analgesia*, 1989: 68: s191.
19. Schwartz AE, et al: Pharmacokinetics and pharmacodynamics of metocurine in the obese. *Anesthesiology*, 1986: 65: A295.
20. Moore FD, et al, "The Body Cell Mass and its Supporting Environment. Body Composition in Health and Disease", published W.B. Saunders Co., U.S.A., 1963, page 166.
21. Kates RE, Leier CV: Dobutamine pharmacokinetics in severe heart failure. *Clinical Pharmacokinetics & Therapeutics*, 1978: 24: 537-541.

Chapter 8

Plasma Protein Binding

Drugs used in anesthesia are all bound to a greater or lesser degree to plasma proteins. Plasma protein binding of drugs has a significant effect on their kinetics and dynamics. Variations of normal physiology and diseases affect both the concentrations and affinity of plasma proteins for drugs. This chapter provides a brief discussion of the relevance of plasma protein drug binding to kinetics and dynamics.

It is first necessary to provide a definition of the term "free fraction". Not all of a drug which is present in the plasma is bound to plasma proteins. The fractional concentration of unbound drug in the plasma is the **free fraction**.

Table 8.1

Physicochemical properties of the three principal plasma proteins which bind drugs.

Protein	Molecular weight (g/mole)	Isoelectric pH
albumin	66,241	4.7
α_1-acid glycoprotein	40,000	2.7
lipoproteins	200,000-3,400,000	?

PROTEIN BINDING AND DRUG DISTRIBUTION

Capillaries and venules of most tissues are relatively impermeable to molecules whose molecular weight is greater than 30,000 g/mole [4]. The plasma proteins to which drugs bind have molecular weights which are greater than 30,000 g/mole. So a drug molecule which is bound to any one of the three plasma proteins listed in table 8.1 cannot readily leave the circulation. The degree to which a given drug can leave the vascular system, and hence tissue drug concentrations achieved by any given dose of that drug, is largely determined by the free fraction of that drug. For any given drug, the distribution volume of that drug is then directly proportional to the free fraction of that drug [1].

The relationship between the free fraction of a given drug and its volume of distribution as measured from the plasma drug concentration is usually derived in the following way [1,9].

The total amount of drug present in the body as measured from the plasma drug concentration is given by equation 8.1.

$$V_d C = V_p C + V_t C_t \qquad (8.1)$$

C is the total plasma drug concentration.
C_t is the total tissue drug concentration.
V_p is the plasma volume.
V_t is the extravascular tissue volume in which the drug is distributed.
V_d is the apparent volume of distribution as measured from the plasma drug concentration.

Divide both sides of equation 8.1 by C to get equation 8.2.

$$V_d = V_p + V_t \frac{C_t}{C} \qquad (8.2)$$

Now the free fraction of drug in the plasma is given by equation 8.3.

$$f_u = \frac{C_u}{C} \qquad (8.3)$$

f_u is the fraction unbound drug in plasma.
C_u is the concentration unbound drug in plasma.

Likewise the tissue free fraction is given by equation 8.4.

$$f_{ut} = \frac{C_{ut}}{C_t} \qquad (8.4)$$

f_{ut} is the fraction unbound drug in extravascular tissues.
C_{ut} is the concentration unbound drug in extravascular tissues.

As it is only free drug that can be exchanged across the capillary, $C_u = C_{ut}$ and so equations 8.3 and 8.4 may be combined to form equation 8.5.

$$\frac{C_t}{C} = \frac{f_u}{f_{ut}} \tag{8.5}$$

Equation 8.5 can now be substituted into equation 8.2 to get equation 8.6. This gives the volume of distribution for a drug with different degrees of tissue and plasma protein binding.

$$V_d = V_p + V_t \frac{f_u}{f_{ut}} \tag{8.6}$$

The plasma drug concentration resulting from administration of a given dose of a drug to such a volume of distribution is given by equation 8.7.

$$C = \frac{\text{Dose}}{V_d} \tag{8.7}$$

Example 8.1 illustrates the effects of differing degrees of plasma protein binding on the volume of distribution, tissue and plasma concentration achieved for a given dose of a drug.

EXAMPLE 8.1:

A 100 mg dose of a very fat insoluble drug is administered to a 70 kg adult. What is the effect of a change of plasma protein drug binding from 90% to 50% on the volume of distribution, and the plasma and tissue drug concentrations achieved with the 100 mg dose? Assume that the tissue binding of this drug is negligible.

Volumes of distribution and free fractions

Very fat insoluble drugs are distributed only within the extracellular fluid volume. This is about 20-25% of the body weight of the average adult. For a 70 kg adult this means an extracellular fluid volume of about 15 liters, made up of 2.5 liters plasma volume and 12.5 liters interstitial fluid volume. So;

- $V_p = 2.5$ L.
- $V_t = 12.5$ L.
- $f_{ut} = 1$ as the tissue binding is negligible.
- $f_u = 0.5$ or 0.1 depending on degree of protein binding, (50% or 90% respectively).

90% plasma protein binding

- Plasma free fraction = f_u = 0.1.
- Using equation 8.6; V_d = 2.5 + 12.5 x (0.1/1) = 3.75 L.
- Total plasma drug concentration after a 100 mg dose = C = 100/3.75 = 26.7 mg/L.
- As the f_{ut} = 1 in this example, plasma free drug concentration = tissue drug concentration = f_u x C = 0.1 x 26.7 = 2.67 mg/L.

50% plasma protein binding

- Plasma free fraction = f_u = 0.5.
- Using equation 8.6; V_d = 2.5 + 12.5 x (0.5/1) = 8.75 L.
- Plasma drug concentration after a 100 mg dose = 100/8.75 = 11.4 mg/L.
- As the f_{ut} = 1 in this example, plasma free drug concentration = tissue drug concentration = f_u x C = 0.5 x 11.4 = 5.7 mg/L.

Effect of change of plasma protein binding

The effect of the change of plasma protein drug binding was twofold.

1. Lowering of the percentage plasma protein binding of a drug caused the distribution volume to increase as less drug remained in the plasma.

2. The total plasma drug concentration achieved for a given dose decreased with a reduction of protein drug binding, but the plasma free drug, and tissue total drug concentrations increased. Increased tissue drug concentration means that the magnitude of the pharmacological effect exerted by that drug increases too.

The relationship between free fraction and drug distribution volume does NOT apply to different drugs. If a drug has a small free fraction, it does not necessarily follow that the distribution volume of that drug will be small. For example, the free fraction of vecuronium = 0.7, while that of fentanyl = 0.16 [1]. However the V_d of fentanyl = 3.8 L/kg, while that of vecuronium = 0.4 L/kg [appendix-A]. Distribution volume is not determined by free fraction alone. Fat solubility, pKa and binding to extracellular tissues also play important roles in determining drug distribution volume [see example 8.2].

EXAMPLE 8.2:

Consider the situation of two drugs, both of which are 90% bound to plasma proteins (f_u = 0.1). The difference between these drugs is that one is very fat soluble with an f_{ut} = 0.03, and the other is very fat insoluble and has an $f_{ut} = 1$. What difference does this difference in fat solubility and tissue binding make to the drug distribution volume in a 70 kg adult?

Fat insoluble drug

Very fat insoluble drugs are distributed only within the extracellular fluid volume. This is about 20-25% of the body weight of the average adult. For a 70 kg adult this means an extracellular fluid volume of about 15 liters, made up of 2.5 liters plasma volume and 12.5 liters interstitial fluid volume. So;

- V_p = 2.5 L.
- V_t = 12.5 L.
- f_u = 0.1.
- f_{ut} = 1.
- Using equation 8.6; V_d = 2.5 + 12.5 x (0.1/1) = 3.75 L.

Fat soluble drug

Fat soluble drugs are distributed within as well as outside cells of the body. For a 70 kg adult this means that with a plasma volume of 2.5 liters, that the drug can distribute throughout all the rest of the body except the bones. Assume a skeletal weight of 10% of body weight, i.e. 7 kg. Therefore the tissue volume throughout which the drug can distribute is about 60.5 kg. So;

- V_p = 2.5 L.
- V_t = 60.5 kg.
- f_u = 0.1.
- f_{ut} = 0.03.
- Using equation 8.6: V_d = 2.5 + 60.5 x (0.1/0.03) = 204.17 L.

Conclusions

It is evident from this example that volume of distribution for different drugs is not only determined by plasma protein binding, but also by the degree of fat solubility or tissue binding.

PROTEIN BINDING AND DRUG CLEARANCE

Most drugs are eliminated by the liver or the kidneys. In order to be eliminated by these organs, a drug must leave the blood to enter them. A drug may enter hepatic and renal tissue by bulk flow, diffusion or active transport.

Protein binding has no effect on the clearance of drugs which enter extravascular tissues by active transport processes. For example, the very rapid renal tubular secretion of some penicillins means that these drugs have a very high renal clearance, despite their very small free fraction [3].

Organ drug clearance differs for drugs with different extraction ratios. A drug may have a "high extraction ratio" or a "low extraction ratio" [see chapter 3].

High extraction ratio drugs

A high extraction ratio drug is removed from the plasma by the organ eliminating that drug regardless of whether the drug is protein bound or not. Such a drug diffuses, or is transported into the organ eliminating that drug at almost the same rate as it enters. The organ clearance of a high extraction ratio drug can be as high as the organ plasma or blood flow. Clearance of such a drug is quite independent of the degree of protein binding [3,1].

Low extraction ratio drugs

The situation is different for low extraction drugs. Protein binding does limit the diffusion rate of such drugs into organs eliminating them. Because of this, the clearance of low extraction ratio drugs is found to be directly related to the degree of protein binding [1,3].

FREE FRACTION AND PHARMACODYNAMICS

Tissue concentrations of a drug are directly proportional to the free fraction of that drug [6, and see example 8.1]. Drug effect is not related to plasma drug concentration, but to drug concentration in the tissue where it is active. So drug effect is directly related to plasma free fraction of a drug [6,8]. Disease, variations of normal physiology and other drugs may alter the free fraction. The percentage change of free fraction induced by these factors is greater for drugs which are normally highly protein bound.

Consider a highly protein bound drug such as alfentanil. Alfentanil is 92% protein bound in the plasma [appendix-B]. A reduction of the percentage binding to 84% means a doubling of the free fraction and hence the plasma free alfentanil concentration. Quite a significant change. The reverse also occurs. If the percentage protein binding of alfentanil increases from 92% to 96%, the free fraction is reduced by a half. This is also a very significant change. Tissue drug concentrations and magnitude of drug effect change accordingly. Clinical investigation has confirmed that changes in protein binding of this order of magnitude can significantly affect the pharmacodynamics of alfentanil [5]. The same is also true for thiopental which is 80-84% protein bound in the plasma [6].

Percentage change of free fraction is less for drugs which are less than 80-85% protein bound. A 10% change in the degree of protein binding has only a minimal effect on the free fraction. Consider the drug pancuronium. Pancuronium is normally only 30% protein bound [appendix-B]. If the percentage binding drops to 20%, or rises to 40%, the free fraction increases or decreases by only 14%. Major clinical effects are unlikely with such relatively small percentage changes of free fraction.

However, regardless of the degree of plasma protein binding, if the percentage change of free fraction is large enough, tissue drug concentrations will change sufficiently to produce a significant clinical effect.

FACTORS AFFECTING PROTEIN DRUG BINDING

Free fraction of a drug may be affected by several factors, both pathological and physiological.

Age

Plasma albumin concentration in persons of age 80 is 12% less than that at age 30 [2]. This may be a part explanation of the slight (about 5%), increase of thiopental free fraction between the ages of 25-80 [7].

α_1-acid glycoprotein concentration in fetuses and neonates is only 33% of that in older children and adults. This is thought to be the cause of the increased free fractions of meperidine, lidocaine and bupivacaine in neonates [1].

Pregnancy

Plasma albumin and α_1-acid glycoprotein concentration are both reduced by pregnancy.

Disease

Plasma albumin concentration is reduced by renal, hepatic, inflammatory and malignant diseases, as well as by cardiac failure and burns [1].

α_1-acid glycoprotein is a protein whose concentration increases in many pathological conditions. Examples of such conditions are chronic pain, burns, trauma, myocardial infarction, and chronic inflammatory diseases such as ulcerative colitis, Crohn's disease and rheumatoid arthritis [1].

Other drugs

It is not uncommon for a person to receive more than one drug at any one time. This is certainly true during anesthesia. It is quite common for a patient to receive as many as 8 different drugs during a single anesthetic. One or more of the drugs administered simultaneously to a patient may compete with other drugs for the same binding sites on plasma proteins. Competition then occurs for these binding sites. This reduces percentage binding of each individual drug below the level that would have occurred were they to have been administered alone.

For example, both thiopental and diazepam bind to plasma albumin. Concurrent administration of drugs which also bind to albumin increases the free fraction of these drugs. Both enflurane, and sulfonamide antibiotics bind to albumin. Concurrent administration of enflurane with diazepam, and of sulfonamides with thiopental significantly increases the free fractions of both diazepam [1] and thiopental [6].

Disease and altered protein binding

Disease states can affect not only plasma protein concentrations, but may also affect the binding of plasma proteins with drugs. The effects of some common disorders will be discussed in subsequent chapters.

CONCLUSIONS

Alterations of plasma protein binding which cause changes in plasma drug free fraction can cause significant changes in drug kinetics and dynamics. This is especially so for drugs with a high degree of protein binding.

In clinical anesthetic practice this means that opiates and hypnotic agents should be administered with caution in patients likely to be hypoproteinemic. The free fractions, and hence the effects of these drugs are likely to be greater than normal.

REFERENCES

1. Wood M: Plasma drug binding: Implications for anesthesiologists. *Anesthesiology*, 1986: 65: 786-804.
2. Dybkaer R, Krakauer R: Relative reference values for clinical chemical and haematological quantities in "healthy" elderly people. *Acta Medica Scandinavica*, 1981: 209: 1-9.
3. Rowland M: Protein binding and drug clearance. *Clinical Pharmacokinetics*, 1984: 9: supplement 1: 10-17.
4. Woerlee GM, "Common Perioperative Problems and the Anaesthetist", published Kluwer Academic Publishers, 1988, ISBN 0-89838-402-8, pages 508-510.
5. Lemmens HJM, et al: Pharmacodynamics of alfentanil: The role of plasma protein binding. *Anesthesiology*, 1989, (submitted for publication)
6. Ghoneim MM, et al: Binding of thiopental to plasma proteins: Effects on distribution in the brain and heart. *Anesthesiology*, 1976: 45: 635-639.
7. Jung D, et al: Thiopental disposition as a function of age in female patients undergoing surgery. *Anesthesiology*, 1982: 56: 263-268.
8. Schuh FT: Influence of haemodilution on the potency of neuromuscular blocking drugs. *British Journal of Anaesthesia*, 1981: 53: 263-265.
9. Rowland M, Tozer TN: "Clinical Pharmacokinetics. Concepts and Applications", published by Lea & Febiger, USA, 1980, ISBN 0-8121-0681-4.

Chapter 9

Cardiac Output

Blood is the medium in which all drugs are transported to and from all tissues of the body. The rate at which blood enters and leaves any tissue is directly related to cardiac output. This means that cardiac output is an important determinant of drug kinetics. Cardiac output changes with age, psychological state, activity level, drugs and disease. This chapter discusses the effects of physiological and pathological changes of cardiac output on the kinetics and dynamics of drugs used in anesthesia.

CIRCULATION TIME AND PRE-RECIRCULATION PHASE

Changes of cardiac output affect both circulation times and pre-recirculation phase drug kinetics.

Pre-recirculation phase

The concept of the pre-recirculation phase has been extensively discussed in chapter 2. In general, the effect of central hemodynamics on pre-recirculation phase drug concentrations is dependant on two main factors. Ejection fractions of the right and left ventricles, and the pulmonary blood volume.

Conditions which increase the ejection fractions of right and left ventricles elevate pre-recirculation phase drug concentrations. Increased ejection fractions occur as a result of tachycardia during physical exertion [5], inotropic and sympathetic nervous stimulation [13], hypovolemia [6] and reduced systemic vascular resistance [7]. The reverse also occurs, pre-recirculation phase drug concentrations decrease when ventricular ejection fractions are reduced.

Conditions which reduce the pulmonary blood volume also increase peak pre-recirculation phase drug concentrations. The anesthesiologically most important cause of reduced pulmonary blood volume is hypovolemia. Hypovolemia reduces pulmonary blood volume as well as increasing the ejection fractions of both ventricles [6], and so increases pre-recirculation phase drug concentrations [8]. Elevation of pulmonary blood volume has the reverse effect, pre-recirculation phase drug concentrations decrease.

The speed with which blood enters the arterial system after intravenous injection, and the duration of the pre-recirculation phase are inversely proportional to the cardiac output [see chapter 2, and also 8,10].

Circulation times

Circulation times between all points in the vascular system are inversely proportional to the cardiac output. So any intravenously administered drug will arrive at any point in the body sooner in a person with a high cardiac output than in a person with a low cardiac output.

DRUG CLEARANCE

Hepatic blood flow is directly proportional to the cardiac output [1,3,4]. The clearances of drugs with a high hepatic extraction ratio such as lidocaine [3], alfentanil [4,9] and indocyanine green [2] are directly proportional to hepatic blood flow and cardiac output.

Because of renal blood flow autoregulation within the normal blood pressure range, renal glomerular filtration rate is not proportional to cardiac output. Therefore it would be expected that the clearances of drugs which are eliminated mainly by the kidneys are not significantly affected by changes of cardiac output. Regrettably the clearances of such drugs have not been studied in relation to the cardiac output, and so this remains only theory.

DRUG DISTRIBUTION AND CARDIAC OUTPUT

Changes of cardiac output and function affect the pre-recirculation and distribution phase drug concentrations of intravenously administered drugs, as well as their distribution volumes.

Anatomy and physiology

Arterial concentrations of an intravenously administered drug are higher than the venous concentrations of the same drug for 2-4 minutes after intravenous bolus administration [21,22]. This is a consequence of the physiology and anatomy of the body. An intravenously administered drug must first pass through the heart and lungs before it can enter the arterial system and finally the organs and tissues of the body. Drug then diffuses into these organs and tissues. If none, or very little of that drug is present in these peripheral tissues, more drug diffuses out of the blood than diffuses back into the blood from these tissues. So the drug concentration in venous blood returning to the heart is initially lower than the arterial concentration of that same drug [18,19,20]. Ultimately sufficient drug diffuses into peripheral tissues so that the rate of drug diffusion out of the blood is the same as the rate of drug diffusion into the blood from all the peripheral tissues. At this point arterial and venous drug concentrations are equal. Venous and arterial blood drug concentrations still continue to decline after this point is achieved because of further diffusion of drug into low-flow tissues and drug elimination. However, the difference between the amount of drug entering and leaving the blood after this point is not large enough to cause a significant arteriovenous drug concentration difference.

The speed with which this process occurs is directly related to the cardiac output, as it is this which determines tissue and organ blood flow.

Distribution phase and cardiac output

The rates of drug redistribution and distribution to tissues are directly related to cardiac output, as it is blood which transports drugs to and from all tissues of the body.

Intercompartmental rate constants and cardiac output

The rate at which a drug is transported to and from any tissue or part of the body is directly proportional to the cardiac output. This means that pharmacokinetic inter-compartmental rate constants are proportional to the cardiac output. This has been confirmed for alfentanil [9], thiopental [10] and lidocaine [16].

Heart failure and drug distribution volumes

Cardiac failure can cause peripheral edema, which increases the extracellular fluid volume. This increases the distribution volumes of fat insoluble drugs, as these drugs are mainly distributed in the extracellular fluid volume. For example, the distribution volume of dobutamine is directly proportional to the degree of peripheral edema [12].

CARDIAC OUTPUT AND DRUG DYNAMICS

Changes of cardiac output affect two aspects of drug dynamics, speed of onset and magnitude of effect.

Speed of onset of drug effect

Circulation times between any two points in the circulation are inversely related to cardiac output [see chapter 2], and it is circulation time which determines the speed with which a drug arrives at any tissue. In addition, the amount of any drug transported to any tissue per unit time is directly related to tissue blood flow, or cardiac output. The actual amount of any given drug entering any tissue is dependant on the extraction ratio of that drug. The kinetics and dynamics of drugs whose rate of entry into a tissue is limited by tissue blood flow rather than the rate of drug diffusion into that tissue, are very sensitive to changes of cardiac output. Rate of onset of effects due to such drugs is directly proportional to cardiac output. Gallamine is an example of a drug where the speed of onset of effect, (muscle relaxation), is directly proportional to the cardiac output [11]. The same is presumably true for many other drugs too [see chapter 2].

Cardiac output is unlikely to affect the speed of onset of drug action of drugs which act by intracellular enzyme induction or inhibition, e.g. the glucocorticoids and theophylline respectively. The same applies to drugs such as insulin [14] which have an extravascular site of action, but diffuse slowly out of blood vessels into their site of action. Rate of onset of effect of such drugs is so slow that recirculation occurs many times before they act. Tissue blood flow will therefore not affect the rate of onset of action of such drugs.

Magnitude and duration of drug effect

As the rate at which many anesthetic drugs diffuse into, and out of tissues is directly proportional to cardiac output, a reduction of cardiac output means that the rate of removal of drugs from tissues is slowed. So after intravenous bolus injection of drugs to persons with a low cardiac output, centrally positioned organs such as heart and brain are exposed for a longer than usual time to relatively high concentrations of drugs during the pre-recirculation and distribution phases. Such persons will develop higher than normal tissue concentrations of drugs in the brain and heart, as a result of which the magnitude and duration of cardiovascular and central nervous system effects resulting from a given drug dose are increased above normal. This has been demonstrated to occur in persons with lower than normal cardiac outputs due to cardiac disease for both the hypnotic [10,17] and cardiovascular effects [17] of thiopental.

The reverse is true for the situation of higher than normal cardiac output.

CLINICAL CONSEQUENCES

The dosages of most drugs administered by anesthesiologists are such that they are mainly effective in the pre-recirculation and distribution phases, and the durations of these phases are inversely proportional to the cardiac output. In addition to this, many intravenous anesthetic drugs have a high or intermediate hepatic extraction, which means that their clearances are directly proportional to the cardiac output. The speed of onset of the effects of drugs such as the muscle relaxants and intravenous hypnotic agents are largely determined by the circulation times as well as tissue blood flow. So cardiac output has a significant effect on the kinetics and dynamics of drugs used in anesthesia. The experienced anesthesiologist appreciates this, and always adjusts anesthetic drug doses and dosage regimens according to his clinical, and entirely qualitative estimation of the "vitality", "health" or "anxiety level" of the patient to whom he administers anesthesia.

REFERENCES

1.   Nies AS, et al: Altered hepatic blood flow and drug disposition. *Clinical Pharmacokinetics*, 1976: 1: 135-155.
2.   Caesar J, et al: The use of indocyanine green in the measurement of hepatic blood flow and as a test of hepatic function. *Clinical Science*, 1961: 21: 43-57.
3.   Stenson RE, et al: Interrelationships of hepatic blood flow, cardiac output, and blood levels of lidocaine in man. *Circulation*, 1971: 43: 205-211.
4.   Chauvin M, et al: The influence of hepatic plasma flow on alfentanil plasma concentration plateaus achieved with an infusion model in humans: Measurement of alfentanil hepatic extraction coefficient. *Anesthesia and Analgesia*, 1986: 65: 999-1003.

5.   Maddahi J, et al: What is the normal range for left and right ejection fraction at different levels of exercise Findings of scintigraphic ventriculography during graded ergometry in 34 normals. *Journal of Nuclear Medicine*, 1980: 21: P5.

6.   Mangano DT, et al: The effect of increasing preload on ventricular output and ejection in man. *Circulation*, 1980: 62: 535-541.

7.   Tsakaris AG, Vandenberg RA: Variations of left ventricular end-diastolic pressure, volume, and ejection fraction with changes in outflow resistance in anesthetized intact dogs. *Circulation Research*, 1968: 23: 213.

8.   Conn HL, Goldberg J: Accuracy of a radiopotassium dilution (Stewart principle) method for the measurement of cardiac output. *Journal of Applied Physiology*, 1955: 7: 542-548.

9.   Krejcie TC, et al: Alfentanil pharmacokinetics: Intravascular space and cardiac output. *Anesthesiology*, 1988: 69: A466.

10.   Christensen JH, et al: Pharmacokinetics and pharmacodynamics of thiopentone. A comparison between young and elderly patients. *Anesthesia*, 1982: 37: 398-404.

11.   Goat VA, et al: The effect of blood flow upon the activity of gallamine triethiodide. *British Journal of Anaesthesia*, 1976: 48: 69-73.

12.   Kates RE, Leier CV: Dobutamine pharmacokinetics in severe heart failure. *Clinical Pharmacology & Therapeutics*, 1978: 24: 537-541.

13.   Slutsky R, et al: Left ventricular size and function after subcutaneous administration of terbutaline. Assessment by cardiac pool imaging. *Chest*, 1981: 79: 501-505.

14.   Sherwin RS, et al: A model of the kinetics of insulin in man. *Journal of Clinical Investigation*, 1974: 53: 1481-1492.

15.   Altman PL, et al (editors), "Handbook of Circulation", pub W.B. Saunders Co., U.S.A., 1959, Library of Congress No. 59-15183, pages 115-124.

16.   Benowitz N, et al: Lidocaine disposition kinetics in monkey and man. II. Effects of hemorrhage and sympathomimetic drug administration. *Clinical Pharmacology & Therapeutics*, 1974: 16: 99-109.

17.   Christensen JH: Increased thiopental sensitivity in cardiac patients. *Acta Anaesthesiologica Scandinavica*, 1985: 29: 702-705.

18.   Price HL, et al: Rates of uptake and release of thiopental by human brain; Relation to kinetics of thiopental anesthesia. *Anesthesiology*, 1957: 18: 171.

19.   Price HL, et al: The uptake of thiopental by body tissues and its relation to the duration of narcosis. *Clinical Pharmacology & Therapeutics*, 1960: 1: 16-22.

20.   Ginsburg JM, Wilde WS: Distribution kinetics of intravenous radiopotassium. *American Journal of Physiology*, 1954: 179: 63-75.

21.   Barratt RL, et al: Kinetics of thiopentone in relation to the site of sampling. *British Journal of Anaesthesia*, 1984: 56: 1385-1391.

22.   Major E, et al: Influence of sample site on blood concentrations of ICI 35 868. *British Journal of Anaesthesia*, 1983: 55: 371-375.

Chapter 10

Age

The aging process causes extensive changes in body composition and function. These changes affect the kinetics and dynamics of drugs used in anesthesia. This chapter will briefly review the consequences of the most important of these changes on the kinetics and dynamics of intravenous drugs used in anesthesia.

PHYSIOLOGICAL AND KINETIC CHANGES DUE TO AGING

In order to understand the effects kinetic and dynamic properties of drugs it is first necessary to briefly review the physiological and structural changes due to aging.

Cardiovascular changes

Blood volume and all body dimensions increase with growth until adulthood. However cardiac index does not increase during growth. This means that the relative blood flow to most organs is unchanged by growth. Because the lengths and volumes of blood vessels does increase, while the cardiac index is unchanged by growth, circulation times between all parts of the body increase with age during growth from child to adult [see table 10.1].

Adult body length, pulmonary and systemic blood volumes do not change much with age. However cardiac index does decrease linearly with age above 30 years [12], and so circulation times between all points in the vascular system increase with age [13].

Changes in liver size and function

Total liver weight and blood flow increase with age after birth until adulthood. The same is not true of liver weight relative to body weight. At birth, the liver is about 5% of body weight, while in the adult it is only 2% of body weight [34]. Hepatic function also changes after birth. Up to 5 months after birth the ability of infants to eliminate drugs by glucuronidation is only about 15-25% of that in adults [28,29]. Other metabolic functions are the same as those in adults, and even if not present at birth, they rapidly develop [28].

Morphine provides a good example of the consequence of the reduced ability to glucuronidate drugs in infants. Elimination of morphine is predominantly by excretion of morphine glucuronide which is synthesized in the liver [30]. Morphine clearance expressed as ml/min/kg, is less in infants younger than 6 months of age than in adults [31].

In adults, liver weight and blood flow both decrease with increasing age. There is a fall of both liver weight and hepatic blood flow of about 18-28% between the ages of 20 to 70 years [31]. Elimination rates of drugs such as antipyrine, imipramine, theophylline and phenytoin are determined by the rate of hepatic metabolism. Clearance of these drugs declines in direct proportion to the reduction of liver mass [31].

Table 10.1.
Changes in body composition and physiology occurring during aging.

AGE (years)	Extracellular fluid volume (% body weight) [3,5,6,7]	Body Fat (% body weight) [4,6,7]	Cardiac Index (L/min/m^2) [12]	Arm-to-lips circulation time (sec) [13]
Birth	39	11	3.4-4	6.5
1	28	21	3.4-4	6.5
10	20-26	20-25	3.4-4	8.5
20-30	20-26	20-30	3.4-4	15.4
40-50	20-26	20-33	2.8-3.2	16.3
60-70	20-26	24-36	2.3-3	17

Changes in renal size and function

The kidneys weigh about 1% of body weight at birth. This declines with growth until they weigh about 0.5% of body weight in adults [34]. Renal blood flow also changes with growth. At birth the kidneys only receive 5-6% of the cardiac output, while adult renal blood flow is about 15-25% of the cardiac output [28].

Glomerular filtration rate increases with age from only 26 ml/1.73 m^2/min at birth, until the adult level of about 120 ml/1.73 m^2/min is achieved at two years of age [14]. The glomerular filtration rate is maximal in healthy young adults of about 20-30 years of age. Renal blood flow achieves adult levels 8 months after birth [28]. This has implications for the clearances of drugs which undergo significant renal elimination. A good example of such a drug is d-tubocurarine, where 63% is excreted unchanged in the urine in a 28 hour period after administration of an intravenous bolus dose to a healthy young adult [32]. Because of the predominantly renal excretion, clearance of d-tubocurarine is lower in the neonate than in the adult, but increases with age in parallel with the increase of glomerular filtration rate [1,33].

Renal function also changes with age in adults. Glomerular filtration rate declines by about 30% in adults between the ages 30 to 80 years [10]. One consequence of this is that the clearances of drugs which are predominantly excreted unchanged in the urine also decrease with age. An example of this is the clearance of d-tubocurarine which is less in the elderly than in the young adult [20].

Table 10.2.

Differences in weight adjusted elimination kinetics of anesthetic drugs in children under two years of age, and adults above 60 years of age, relative to healthy young adults.

DRUG	INFANTS (< 2 years)			AGED ADULTS (> 60 years)		
	V_d	Cl	$t_{1/2\beta}$	V_d	Cl	$t_{1/2\beta}$
Thiopental				↑[11]	0	↑
Etomidate				0[15]	↓	↑
Atropine	↑[16]	0	↑	0[16]	↓	↑
Fentanyl	0[17]	↑	↓	0[18]	↓	↑
Alfentanil				0[19]	↓	↑
d-Tubocurarine	↑[1]	0	↑	↓[20]	↓	↑
Pancuronium				0[21]	↓	↑
Vecuronium	↑[2]	0	0	↓[22]	↓	0
Atracurium	↑[8]	↑	0	↑[23]	↑	↑

↑ increased above value in normal young adult.
↓ decreased below value in normal young adult.
0 no change from value in normal young adult.

Plasma drug binding proteins and age

The plasma concentrations of drug binding proteins also change with age. Albumin concentration decreases [10], and α_1-acid glycoprotein concentration increases with age [9]. However these age related changes in plasma protein concentrations are not large. So their effect on plasma protein binding of anesthetic drugs is also not large. These changes therefore only affect drugs whose percentage plasma protein binding is greater than 85-90% [9].

CONSEQUENCES OF CHANGED DRUG KINETICS AND DYNAMICS

Age related changes in drug kinetics and dynamics have consequences for anesthetic drug dosage and dosage regimens.

Induction agents

An effective hypnotic dose of an induction agent injected as an intravenous bolus takes longer to induce hypnosis in an elderly than in a young person. In addition to this, the dose required to induce hypnosis in an elderly person is less than in a younger person [11,15,24]. However, aging does not change the $t_{1/2}k_{eo}$ or the concentration-effect curves of induction agents [15, 25]. This means that the MEC for hypnosis, and the speed with which a given plasma drug concentration exerts an effect is also unchanged by age.

The reason for the slower onset of hypnosis, and the requirement for a lower induction dose in the elderly lies in age induced physiological changes.

- Cardiac output decreases, and so all circulation times increase with age [table 10.1]. So the older the person, the longer it takes for any intravenously administered induction agent to arrive in the brain and induce hypnosis.

- All intravenous anesthetic induction agents induce their effects in the pre-recirculation phase [see chapters 2 and 5]. Pre-recirculation phase drug kinetics are changed by the aging process. Cardiac index is lower in the elderly adult than in the child or the younger adult, due to a reduction of average pulse rate, stroke volume and ventricular ejection fractions, while the pulmonary blood volume is relatively unchanged [12]. Reduced cardiac output means that the onset of the pre-recirculation phase peak concentration is delayed, and the duration of the pre-recirculation phase prolonged in the elderly. In addition the reduced cardiac output together with decreased ventricular ejection fractions, and unchanged pulmonary blood volume means that the peak pre-recirculation phase drug concentration is somewhat lower in the elderly than in the younger adult, (k_p, k_L, and k_R all decrease) [see chapter 2]. Prolongation of the pre-recirculation phase means that the relatively high pre-recirculation phase drug concentrations remain for a longer time in elderly than in younger persons. So the time available for action is longer and the effects more profound in the elderly. In the case of anesthetic induction agents this all means that the time to onset of hypnosis due to intravenous induction agents increases with increasing age, and the hypnotic and myocardial depressant effects of a given dose are more profound and last longer [see simulation in figure 10.1].

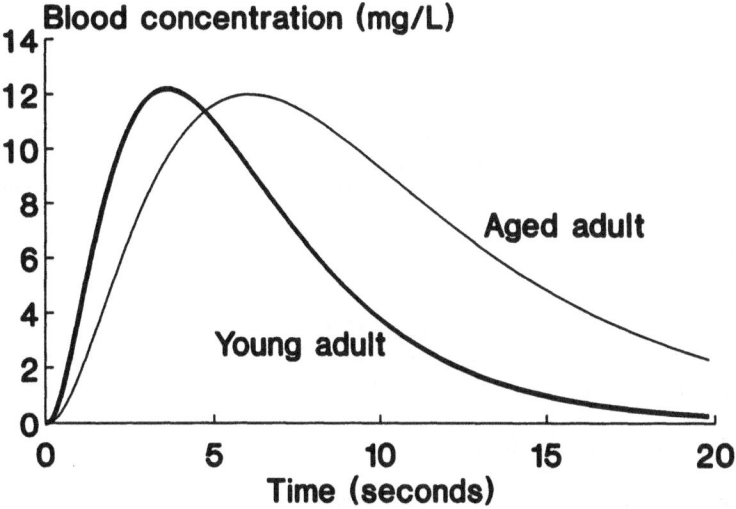

Figure 10.1: The effect of aging on pre-recirculation phase kinetics of 10 mg of a drug administered as a rapid intravenous bolus. Data for calculating k_R, k_p, and k_L are from Brandfonbrener et al (1955) [12]. Peak concentration is lower in the aged than in younger adults, and the plasma drug concentrations remain higher for a longer time.

Opiates

Opiate requirements are also reduced in the elderly. However opiate pharmacodynamics are unchanged by age in adults. This has been best investigated for alfentanil, where it has been shown that the plasma alfentanil concentrations required in adults to suppress hemodynamic responses to various stimuli are unchanged by age [26]. The effect of aging in adults is to reduce opiate clearance and so prolong elimination half life, but not to change the MEC for any effect. This means that aged adults require the same opiate dosages as younger adults to achieve the same effect. However subsequent dosage intervals should be longer because of prolongation of elimination half lives.

Opiate pharmacodynamics have not been extensively investigated in children, and very little information is available on the subject.

Non-depolarizing muscle relaxants

Not only do the kinetics of non-depolarizing muscle relaxants differ in different age groups, but the pharmacodynamic properties also differ. This has been well studied for several relaxants. The effect of aging on the kinetics of these drugs is shown by table 10.2. In the infant of less than 2 years of age, the relatively high extracellular fluid volume means that weight adjusted distribution volumes are larger than in adults [table 7.3]. However non-depolarizing relaxant clearance is the same in infants as in young adults, and so elimination half lives of these drugs are longer in infants [see equation 3.28].

Clearances of non-depolarizing relaxants are lower in the elderly than in the young adult. So elimination half lives of non-depolarizing relaxants increase with age in adults. The MEC for differing degrees of muscle relaxation for any given relaxant differs in different age groups, but the $t_{1/2}k_{eo}$ does not vary with age [1,2]. The two best studied drugs are vecuronium and d-tubocurarine [see table 10.3].

Table 10.3.

The table lists $t_{1/2}k_{eo}$ values, and average muscle relaxant concentrations at which muscle strength is reduced by 50% (EC_{50}) in different age groups for d-tubocurarine [1] and vecuronium [2]. The dose of each drug required to produce this degree of relaxation (D_{50}) is also compared for these two relaxants.

AGE GROUP	Vecuronium			d-Tubocurarine		
	$t_{1/2}k_{eo}$ (min)	EC_{50} (μg/L)	D_{50} (mg/kg)	$t_{1/2}k_{eo}$ (min)	EC_{50} (mg/L)	D_{50} (mg/kg)
Neonates (0-2 months)				6.3	0.18	0.155
Infants (2 months - 1 year)	3.9	0.057	0.021	7.5	0.27	0.158
Adults (12 years +)	3.7	0.094	0.025	6.8	0.53	0.152

Table 10.3 shows that infants are more sensitive than adults to a given plasma concentration of non-depolarizing muscle relaxants. However, as weight adjusted distribution volumes of non-depolarizing relaxants are larger in infants [table 7.3], the doses required to produce the same effects in infants and adults are the same [tables 10.2 and 10.3]. This does not mean that the duration of action of these muscle relaxants is the same in infants and adults. Elimination half lives of non-depolarizing relaxants are longer in infants than in adults [table 10.2]. So while the dose required for a given effect may be the same, the duration of action is longer in infants than in adults [see figure 10.2].

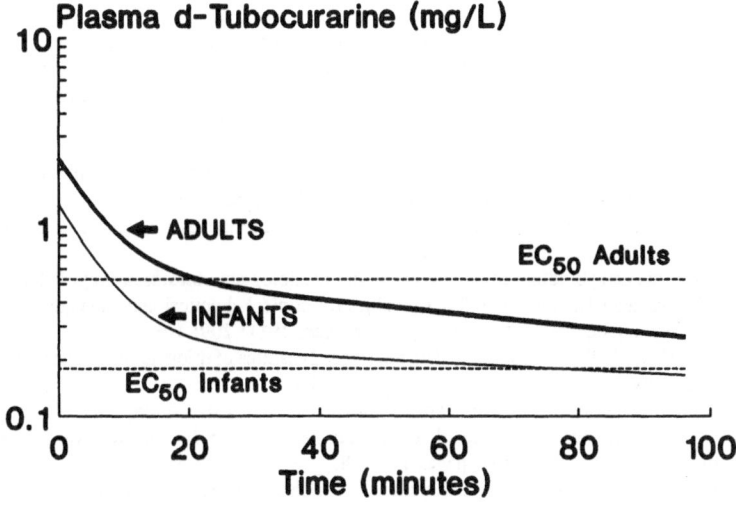

Figure 10.2: Plasma concentration-time curves of a 0.5 mg/kg dose of d-tubocurarine administered to infants and adults shown relative to the EC_{50} for d-tubocurarine in these two age groups. A given dose of d-tubocurarine will exert a longer-lasting effect in infants than in adults.

CONCLUSIONS

The extensive changes in body physiology and composition due to aging have a significant effect on drug kinetics and dynamics at the two extremes of life. These changes must be taken into account whenever anesthetic drugs are administered to patients at either age extreme.

REFERENCES

1. Fisher DM, et al: Pharmacokinetics and pharmacodynamics of d-tubocurarine in infants, children, and adults. *Anesthesiology*, 1982: 57: 203-208.
2. Fisher DM, et al: Vecuronium kinetics and dynamics in anesthetized infants and children. *Clinical Pharmacology & Therapeutics*, 1985: 37: 402-406.
3. Friis-Hansen B: Body water compartments in children: Changes during growth and related changes in body composition. *Pediatrics*, 1961: 28: 169-181.

4. Friis-Hansen B: Body composition during growth. In vivo measurements and biochemical data correlated to differential anatomical growth. *Pediatrics*, 1971: 47: 264-274.
5. Skrabal F, et al: Equations for the prediction of normal values for exchangeable sodium, exchangeable potassium, extracellular volume, and total body water. *British Medical Journal*, 1973 2: 37-38.
6. Bruce A, et al: Prediction of normal body potassium, body water and body fat in adults on the basis of body height, body weight and age. *Scandinavian Journal of Clinical & Laboratory Investigation*, 1980: 40: 461-463.
7. Moore FD, et al, "The Body Cell Mass and its Supporting Environment. Body Composition in Health and Disease", published W.B. Saunders Co., U.S.A., 1963, page 166.
8. Brandom BW, et al: Pharmacokinetics of atracurium in anesthetized infants and children. *British Journal of Anaesthesia*, 1986: 58: 1210-1213.
9. Wood M: Plasma drug binding: Implications for anesthesiologists. *Anesthesiology*, 1986: 65: 786-804.
10. Dybkaer R, Krakauer R: Relative reference values for clinical chemical and haematological quantities in "healthy" elderly people. *Acta Medica Scandinavica*, 1981: 209: 1-9.
11. Christensen JH, et al: Pharmacokinetics and pharmacodynamics of thiopentone. A comparison between young and elderly patients. *Anesthesia*, 1982: 37: 398-404.
12. Brandfonbrener M, et al: Changes in cardiac output with age. *Circulation*, 1955: 12: 557-566.
13. Altman PL, et al (editors), "Handbook of Circulation", pub W.B. Saunders Co., U.S.A., 1959, Library of Congress No. 59-15183, pages 115-118.
14. Rubin MI, et al: Maturation of renal function in childhood; Clearance studies. *Journal of Clinical Investigation*, 1949: 28: 1144.
15. Arden J, et al: Increased sensitivity to etomidate in the elderly: Initial distribution versus altered brain response. *Anesthesiology*, 1986: 65: 19-27.
16. Virtanen R, et al: Pharmacokinetic studies on atropine with special reference to age. *Acta Anaesthesiologica Scandinavica*, 1982: 26: 297-300.
17. Singleton MA, et al: Pharmacokinetics of fentanyl for infants and adults. *Anesthesiology*, 1984: 61: A440.
18. Bentley JB, et al: Age and fentanyl pharmacokinetics. *Anesthesia and Analgesia*, 1982: 61: 968-971.
19. Lemmens HJM et al: Influence of age on the pharmacokinetics of alfentanil. *Anesthesiology*, 1988: 69: A629.
20. Matteo RS, et al: Pharmacokinetics of d-tubocurarine in the aged. *Anesthesiology*, 1982: 57: A271.
21. Duvaldestin P, et al: Pharmacokinetics, pharmacodynamics, and dose-response relationships of pancuronium in control and elderly subjects. *Anesthesiology*, 1982: 56: 36-40.
22. Rupp SM, et al: Pharmacokinetics and pharmacodynamics of vecuronium in the elderly. *Anesthesiology*, 1983: 59: A270.
23. Kitts JB, et al: Pharmacokinetics of atracurium in elderly and young adults. *Anesthesiology*, 1988: 69: A482.
24. Homer TD, Stanski DR: The effect of increasing age on thiopental and anesthetic requirement. *Anesthesiology*, 1985: 62: 714-724.
25. Homer TD, Stanski DR: The effect of increasing age on thiopental disposition and anesthetic requirement. *Anesthesiology*, 1985: 62: 714-724.
26. Lemmens HJM, et al: Age has no effect on the pharmacodynamics of alfentanil. *Anesthesia and Analgesia*, 1988: 67: 956-960.
27. Olkkola KT, et al: Kinetics and dynamics of postoperative intravenous morphine in children. *Clinical Pharmacology & Therapeutics*, 1988: 44: 128-135.
28. Besunder JB, et al: Principles of drug biodisposition in the neonate. A critical evaluation of the pharmacokinetic-pharmacodynamic interface. (Part I). *Clinical Pharmacokinetics*, 1988: 14: 189-216.
29. Morselli PL: Clinical pharmacokinetics in neonates. *Clinical Pharmacokinetics*, 1976: 1: 81-98.

30. Patwardhan RV, et al: Normal metabolism of morphine in cirrhosis. *Gastroenterology*, 1981: 81: 1006-1011.
31. Woodhouse KW, Wynne HA: Age-related changes in liver size and hepatic blood flow. The influence on drug metabolism in the elderly. *Clinical Pharmacokinetics*, 1988: 15: 287-294.
32. Meijer DKF, et al: Comparative pharmacokinetics of d-tubocurarine and metocurine in man. *Anesthesiology*, 1979: 51: 402-407.
33. Matteo RS, et al: Pharmacokinetics of d-tubocurarine in neonates, infants and children. *Anesthesiology*, 1982: 57: A269.
34. Diem K, Lentner C, (editors), "Wissenschaftliche Tabellen", 7th edition, published CIBA-GEIGY, Basel, 1968, page 515.

Chapter 11

Obesity

Obesity is an example of an extreme variation of body composition. The physiological changes induced by obesity present the anesthesiologist with many perioperative problems [7], in addition to which these changes also affect the pharmacology of anesthetic drugs.

A person is defined as obese when their body weight is 20% greater than their ideal body weight [8].

$$IdealWeight(kg) - 0.9 \times [BodyLength(cm) - 100] \tag{11.1}$$

PHYSIOLOGICAL AND KINETIC CHANGES DUE TO OBESITY

Obesity induces several changes in physiology which affect drug kinetics. These will be briefly discussed.

Increased total body fat content

A normal young adult has a total body fat content which varies between 15-26% of body weight, while an obese adult may have a total body fat content which is as much as 60% of body weight. This is because both adipocyte number and fat content are increased in obese persons [9]. Consequently the weight adjusted distribution volumes of fat-soluble drugs are increased in obesity. An example of this is shown in table 7.4 for thiopental.

Extracellular fluid volume

The interstitial fluid volume of adipose tissue is about the same as that of muscle tissue, but slightly less than that of the body as a whole [table 2.3]. This means that the weight adjusted extracellular fluid volume of an obese person is only slightly less than that of a non-obese person

[1,2,6]. Therefore the weight adjusted distribution volumes of relatively fat-insoluble drugs are unchanged by obesity. An example of this is shown in table 7.5 for vecuronium.

Increased cardiac output

Adipose tissue has a blood flow of 20-70 ml/kg/min [table 2.3]. So if body weight is increased by 20 kg adipose tissue, the cardiac output would increase by 0.4-1.4 L/min. Clinical investigation has confirmed that the cardiac output is increased above normal in obesity. The cardiac output of a grossly obese adult with a body weight as much as 100 kg above ideal body weight may be as high as 10 L/min [8]. Increased cardiac output affects pre-recirculation phase drug kinetics [see chapter 2].

Obesity and renal function

Glomerular filtration rate is directly proportional to body weight. The capacities of some renal tubular drug secretory processes also increase in obesity. Examples of this are provided by the renal clearances of procainamide and cimetidine which are increased in obese persons [10].

Obesity and hepatic function

Obesity also affects the ability of the liver to metabolize drugs. The rate at which the liver can conjugate, (e.g. glucuronate) drugs is increased, while hepatic drug oxidation and acetylation rates are unchanged in obese adults [10].

EFFECTS OF OBESITY ON KINETICS OF ANESTHETIC DRUGS

Altered body composition, increased weight, and changes in renal and hepatic function, mean that obesity changes the kinetics of drugs used in anesthesia [see table 11.1]. The reasons for the rather diverse changes of kinetic properties shown in table 11.1 vary. Obesity increases the weight adjusted distribution volumes of fat-soluble drugs such as thiopental, midazolam and propofol. This is because the percentage body fat is increased in obesity. The weight adjusted distribution volume of alfentanil is not increased by obesity. This latter is to be expected as alfentanil is not very fat-soluble [see appendix-B]. Curiously, the distribution volume of fentanyl is not increased in obesity. This is surprising as fentanyl is a very fat-soluble drug. The percentage extracellular fluid volume is relatively normal in obese persons. So weight adjusted distribution volumes of the non-depolarizing muscle relaxants are unchanged by obesity.

Changes of weight adjusted drug clearance due to obesity are more difficult to explain. Total and weight adjusted clearances of vecuronium [4] and metocurine [5] are reduced below normal by obesity. This is unexpected as both drugs undergo significant renal and hepatic excretion as unchanged drug [tables 13.1 and 14.1]. Obesity increases glomerular filtration rate, although it does not affect hepatic blood flow, and so the clearances of these two relaxants would most likely increase. The increased weight adjusted clearance of thiopental is equally unexpected. Thiopental undergoes extensive oxidative metabolism in the liver, and only 0.3% of a single dose of thiopental is excreted unchanged in the urine in 24 hours [15]. As obesity does not affect the rate of oxidative drug metabolism [10], the clearance of thiopental would most likely be unchanged. So the explanation for the increased clearance of thiopental is unclear. Likewise, the causes for the lack of change of fentanyl and midazolam clearances, and the reduced clearance of alfentanil are also unclear.

In general the final common effect of obesity is to prolong the elimination half lives of many drugs used in anesthesia.

Table 11.1.
Effect of obesity on the weight adjusted elimination kinetics of some drugs used in anesthesia.

DRUG	V_d (L/kg)	Cl (L/kg/h)	$t_{1/2\beta}$ (min)
Thiopental [3]	↑	↑	↑
Propofol [11]	↑	↑	0
Midazolam [12]	↑	0	↑
Fentanyl [13]	0	0	0
Alfentanil [14]	0	↓	↑
Metocurine [5]	0	↓	↑
Vecuronium [4]	0	↓	↑

↑ = increased above the level in normal adults.
↓ = decreased below the level in normal adults.
0 = no different from the level in normal adults.

CLINICAL CONSEQUENCES

Obesity affects the dosages and dosage regimens of intravenous anesthetic drugs.

Induction agents

Induction agents are administered in doses which are usually sufficient to induce hypnosis within 20-45 seconds. Therefore these drugs induce hypnosis in the pre-recirculation phase [see chapter 2], and speed of onset of hypnosis due to these drugs is dependant on cardiac output, right and left ventricular ejection fractions, and pulmonary blood volume.

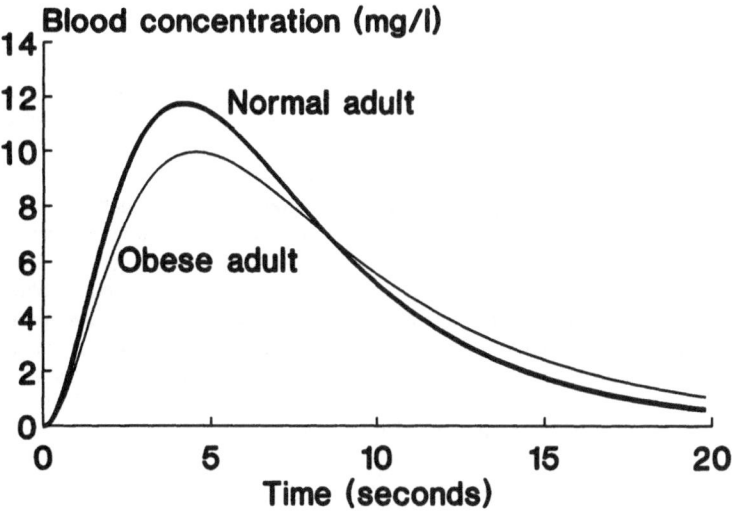

Figure 11.1: Cardiac output and pulmonary blood volume are increased in the obese adult. Pulmonary blood volume is increased to a greater degree than the cardiac output. Ventricular ejection fractions are usually unchanged. The consequences of these changes on the pre-recirculation phase are simulated here for a rapidly administered 10 mg intravenous bolus dose of a drug.

The TOTAL hypnotic dose of an intravenous induction agent such as thiopental required to induce hypnosis in obese adults is larger than in non-obese adults [3,16]. Changes in central hemodynamics induced by obesity are the cause of this. Cardiac output [17,18,19], total blood volume, and pulmonary blood volume [18] are increased in obese adults. Pulmonary blood volume in obese adults may be as much as 50% greater than in normal adults [19]. Elevation of the cardiac output occurs without an increase of heart rate, because stoke volume is increased due to ventricular dilation together with maintenance of normal ejection fractions of both ventricles [17,18]. It is only in very morbidly obese persons that cardiac function is depressed and ejection fractions are reduced below normal [17,18]. However, regardless of cardiac function, cardiac output never increases to the same degree as the pulmonary blood volume [19], and it is this which is the major effect of obesity on pre-recirculation phase kinetics. A relative increase of pulmonary blood volume reduces peak pre-recirculation phase drug concentrations, (k_R, and k_L, are unchanged, reduced k_p) [see chapter 2]. The result of these changes is that obese persons require a larger than usual dose of anesthetic induction agents to induce hypnosis.

Drugs acting within the V_c or V_d

With the exception of the intravenous induction agents, all anesthetic drugs continue to be pharmacologically active while distributed throughout the V_c and V_d. This means that they act while being distributed, redistributed and eliminated from the V_c and V_d. Obesity induced changes in drug elimination kinetics have consequences for the clinician. The consequences of these changes must be considered separately for fat-soluble and fat-insoluble drugs.

Because the relative interstitial fluid volume of adipose tissue is much the same as that of muscle, weight adjusted distribution volumes of fat-insoluble drugs such as muscle relaxants are relatively unchanged by obesity. So weight adjusted dosages of these drugs are also unchanged. However elimination half lives of these drugs may be increased or decreased by obesity induced changes in drug clearance. This means that dosage interval must be adjusted accordingly.

Weight adjusted distribution volumes of fat-soluble drugs such as benzodiazepines are increased by obesity [table 11.1]. So the dosages required of such drugs, expressed as mg/kg, may need to be higher than in non-obese adults. Lengthening of elimination half lives of fat-soluble drugs mean that their dosage intervals must also be increased accordingly.

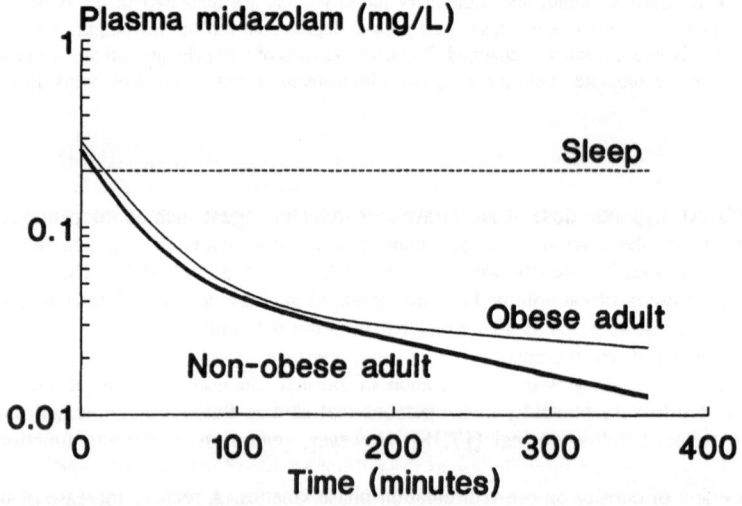

Figure 11.2: Plasma concentration-time curves of a 0.15 mg/kg dose of midazolam administered to obese and non-obese adults. Midazolam is a fat soluble drug. The increased V_d in obese adults results in a longer $t_{1/2\beta}$ than in non-obese adults.

EXAMPLE 11.1:

Midazolam is an example of a fat soluble drug. Obesity causes the weight adjusted V_d to increase, but weight adjusted clearance is unchanged. The effect of these changes is to lengthen the elimination half [equation 3.28].

Consider the effects of intravenous bolus administration of 0.15 mg/kg midazolam to obese and normal adults. Kinetic data used in this example are from Greenblatt et al (1984) [12], and this example has also been simulated in figure 11.2.

	Non-obese	Obese
Dose (mg/kg)	0.15	0.15
MEC (hypnosis) (mg/L)	0.2	0.2
$t_{1/2\alpha}$ (minutes)	18.6	24
$t_{1/2\beta}$ (minutes)	164	504
A_x (kg/L)	1.35	1.68
B_x (kg/L)	0.38	0.25
A = dose x A_x (mg/L)	0.203	0.252
B = dose x B_x (mg/L)	0.057	0.038
C (mg/L) at time = 0 min	0.26	0.29
C (mg/L) at time = 1 x $t_{1/2\alpha}$	0.154 < MEC	0.162 < MEC

These calculations show that the practical consequences of obesity on the clinical use of this dose of midazolam are negligible. Hypnosis is terminated in both obese and non-obese adults by drug redistribution within a time less than one $t_{1/2\alpha}$. Figure 11.2 does show that obesity will prolong the effects of higher doses because of obesity induced prolongation of the elimination half life.

REFERENCES

1. Skrabal F, et al: Equations for the prediction of normal values for exchangeable sodium, exchangeable potassium, extracellular volume, and total body water. *British Medical Journal*, 1973 2: 37-38.
2. Bruce A, et al: Prediction of normal body potassium, body water and body fat in adults on the basis of body height, body weight and age. *Scandinavian Journal of Clinical & Laboratory Investigation*, 1980: 40: 461-463.

3.   Jung D, et al: Thiopental disposition in lean and obese patients undergoing surgery. *Anesthesiology*, 1982: 56: 269-274.

4.   Matteo RS, et al: Pharmacokinetics and pharmacodynamics of vecuronium in the obese surgical patient. *Anesthesia and Analgesia*, 1989: 68: s191.

5.   Schwartz AE, et al: Pharmacokinetics and pharmacodynamics of metocurine in the obese. *Anesthesiology*, 1986: 65: A295.

6.   Moore FD, et al, "The Body Cell Mass and its Supporting Environment. Body Composition in Health and Disease", published W.B. Saunders Co., U.S.A., 1963, page 166.

7.   Fisher A, et al: Obesity: Its relation to anaesthesia. *Anaesthesia*, 1975: 30: 633-647.

8.   Abernathy DR, Greenblatt DJ: Pharmacokinetics of drugs in obesity. *Clinical Pharmacokinetics*, 1982: 7: 108-124.

9.   Hirsch J, Batchelor B: Adipose tissue cellularity in human obesity. *Clinics in Endocrinology and Metabolism*, 1976: 5: 299-311.

10.   Abernathy DR, Greenblatt DJ: Drug disposition in obese humans. An update. *Clinical Pharmacokinetics*, 1986: 11: 199-213.

11.   Servin F, et al: Propofol pharmacokinetics in morbidly obese patients. *Anesthesiology*, 1988: 69: A463.

12.   Greenblatt DJ, et al: Effect of age, gender, and obesity on midazolam kinetics. *Anesthesiology*, 1984: 61: 27-35.

13.   Bentley JB, et al: Fentanyl pharmacokinetics in obese and nonobese patients. *Anesthesiology*, 1981: 55: A177.

14.   Bentley JB, et al: Obesity and alfentanil pharmacokinetics. *Anesthesia and Analgesia*, 1983: 62: 251.

15.   Greene NM: The metabolism of drugs employed in anesthesia. Part II. *Anesthesiology*, 1968: 29: 327.

16.   Cork RC, et al: General anesthesia for morbidly obese patients - An examination of postoperative outcomes. *Anesthesiology*, 1981: 54: 310-313.

17.   De Devitiis O, et al: Obesity and cardiac function. *Circulation*, 1981: 64: 477-482.

18.   Messerli FH: Cardiovascular effects of obesity and hypertension. *Lancet*, 1982: 1: 1165-1168.

19.   Rochester DF, Enson Y: Current concepts in the pathogenesis of the obesity-hypoventilation syndrome. Mechanical and circulatory factors. *American Journal of Medicine*, 1974: 57: 402-420.

Chapter 12

Pregnancy Related Problems

Pregnancy and birth present the anesthesiologist with a variety of unique problems. Anesthetic drugs administered to a pregnant woman will not only affect the woman, but may also affect the child too. It is for this reason that this chapter is divided into two parts. The first part is a brief review of the effects of pregnancy on the kinetics and dynamics of intravenously administered drugs used in anesthesia. The second part is a discussion of the effects of these same drugs on the infant delivered by caesarean section.

PREGNANCY

Pregnancy causes profound changes in female physiology and anatomy. These changes are capable of altering the kinetics of drugs used in anesthesia. However, relatively few studies have been made on the kinetics of anesthetic drugs during pregnancy. The main reason for this is undoubtedly the fact that most pregnant women are very healthy. They rarely require the attentions of an anesthesiologist except during labor and caesarean section. So most studies on the kinetics of anesthetic drugs during pregnancy have been done using women undergoing caesarean section.

Physiological alterations due to pregnancy

Many studies have been made of the changes in maternal physiology during pregnancy, and these changes have direct relevance to the kinetics of the drugs administered.

- Total body fat is increased by up to 20-40% above non-pregnant content.
- Extracellular fluid volume is increased above normal.
- Plasma volume increases by up to 50% above the non-pregnant level, most of the increase having occurred by 24 weeks, thereafter increasing slowly until term [1].

- Red cell volume increases by 20% during pregnancy [1]. This is less than the 50% increase of plasma volume. As a result most pregnant women have a mild dilutional anemia.
- Both the increased red cell and plasma volume mean that the blood volume also increases during pregnancy by up to 40% above non-pregnant levels [1]
- Cardiac output increases by up to 27-64% above non-pregnant levels, the increase being maximal in the third trimester [2]. These changes are secondary to the increased blood volume, as well as the changes in cardiovascular and neuro-endocrine function during pregnancy. After 36 weeks, the weight of the fetus may cause significant inferior vena cava compression when the mother lies in the supine position. This may reduce the cardiac output to such a degree that this position becomes impossible at this time [2,4].
- Increased cardiac output means that all circulation times are reduced [6].
- During labor the cardiac output increases even further, mainly due to pain and anxiety. Furthermore, about 250 ml of blood is also expelled from the uterus during each uterine contraction. During a uterine contraction the cardiac output may increase by up to 30% above the level between contractions [3].
- Liver blood flow does not increase significantly during pregnancy [5].
- Glomerular filtration rate increases by up to 50% above non-pregnant levels by 16 weeks, and remains at this level until the end of pregnancy.

Effect of pregnancy on drug kinetics

Increased total body fat and water, in addition to increased cardiac output as well as glomerular filtration rate may all be expected to affect the kinetics of intravenous anesthetic drugs. The few studies performed confirm this [see table 12.1]. However the results of these studies are not in any way consistent. Increased extracellular fluid volume and total body fat content may be expected to increase the weight adjusted distribution volumes of all drugs, and this does not occur. Increased renal clearance of some drugs does reduce their elimination half lives, but this is again not always a consistent finding.

Drug dynamics and pregnancy

Cardiac output is increased in pregnancy. This decreases circulation times between all points of the circulation [6], reducing arrival and onset times of all intravenously administered drugs. Consider the arm-to-brain circulation time. This decreases with increasing duration of gestation, and the anesthetist can expect the hypnotic effect of a sleep dose of thiopental to occur sooner in pregnant women than in non-pregnant women.

The effect of pregnancy on the plasma concentration-effect relationships of drugs used in anesthesia has not been extensively investigated.

Table 12.1.
Effects of pregnancy on the kinetics of several intravenously administered drugs.

Drug	V_d	Cl	$t_{1/2\beta}$
Thiopental [7]	↑	0/↑	↑
Meperidine [8,9]	0	0	0
Pancuronium [10,11]	0	↑	↓
Vecuronium [11]	↓	0/↑	↓

↑ increased above value in nonpregnant woman.
↓ decreased below value in nonpregnant woman.
0 no change.

THE NEWBORN AND CAESAREAN SECTION

Drugs administered to the mother to provide anaesthesia during caesarean section may cross the placental barrier and enter the newborn baby. The anesthesiologist is therefore faced with a dilemma. A woman undergoing caesarean section must be anesthetized, but the newly born baby must be viable immediately after delivery. The latter means that the baby must not be significantly affected by anesthetic drugs which at the time of delivery are still present in sufficient concentrations in maternal tissues so that the mother is anesthetized.

It is the anesthesiologist who must decide which drugs to use to provide anesthesia for the mother so as to satisfy these two different purposes. Any decision to use any particular anesthetic drug must be based on knowledge of the ability of that drug to cross the placental barrier and affect the newborn baby. Such a decision is based on known fetal/maternal plasma concentration ratios of anesthetic drugs.

Table 12.2.
Fetal/Maternal (F/M) plasma concentration ratios of various anesthetic drugs
measured at delivery, 5-15 minutes after
intravenous bolus administration of the
drugs to the mothers.

DRUG	F/M
Thiopental [7,12]	1.1
Diazepam [12]	1.2
Meperidine [8,12]	1-1.1
Alfentanil [12]	0.4
Sufentanil [12]	0.52
Alcuronium [14]	0.18
Pancuronium [10,11]	0.19
Vecuronium [11]	0.11
Atracurium [17]	0.12
Atropine [12,15]	0.5-1.2

Fetal/Maternal concentration ratio

There is a body of data on the fetal/maternal (F/M) plasma concentration ratios of various drugs [12]. This data is derived from drug concentration measurements in maternal venous blood, and umbilical venous blood, sampled at the time of delivery of infants by caesarean section. The usual time of sampling in nearly all studies is 5-15 minutes after intravenous bolus administration of the drug concerned to the woman undergoing caesarean section. Five to fifteen minutes is the usual time taken to deliver a baby by caesarean section after induction of anesthesia. So such data are very relevant for clinical decision making purposes. F/M plasma concentration ratios of a number of drugs used in anesthesia are listed in table 12.2.

Clinical consequences of placental drug transfer

The neonatal effects of any anesthetic drug administered to a woman undergoing caesarean section are dependant on the amount of that drug which has entered the baby prior to clamping the umbilical cord, and the magnitude of the neonatal plasma drug concentration at the time the umbilical cord is clamped.

Induction agents

Available data indicate that intravenously administered hypnotic drugs freely cross the placental barrrier [12, and table 12.2]. Therefore fetal plasma concentrations of these drugs most likely parallel those in the mother. The pharmacodynamics of intravenous hypnotic drugs have not been studied in neonates. However extensive clinical experience has shown that babies are nearly always active and awake when delivered by caesarean section 5-15 minutes after their mothers have been administered intravenous hypnotic drugs to induce general anesthesia. This latter empirical fact lends some support for the idea that the neonatal effects of these drugs parallel those in the mother, even though the pharmacodynamics of these drugs may differ between adults and neonates.

Opiates

Opiates readily cross the placental barrier to enter the fetal circulation. Experience has shown that normal clinical doses of opiates all cause significant respiratory depression in newly born infants. It is for this reason that anesthesiologists avoid the administration of these drugs to women undergoing caesarean section until after the baby has been delivered.

Muscle relaxants

Use of suxamethonium, a depolarizing neuromuscular junction blocking drug, has never been shown to cause significant neonatal muscle paralysis. This is to be expected as a baby is never delivered before 5-15 minutes has passed after intravenous bolus administration, and suxamethonium is completely eliminated by this time.

However the non-depolarizing muscle relaxants are not eliminated within 5-15 minutes after intravenous bolus administration. These drugs also cross the placenta to a limited degree, and neonates are more sensitive to the muscle relaxant effects of these drugs than are adults. Fortunately, extensive clinical experience, and studies of non-depolarizing muscle relaxants have shown that administration of normal clinical doses of non-depolarizing muscle relaxant drugs to provide muscle relaxation during caesarean section does not cause significant neonatal hypotonia, muscle paralysis, or respiratory depression [10,11]. So these drugs may be administered during anesthesia for caesarean section prior to delivery of the baby. This can also be predicted using known kinetic and dynamic data for non-depolarizing relaxants [see example 12.1]

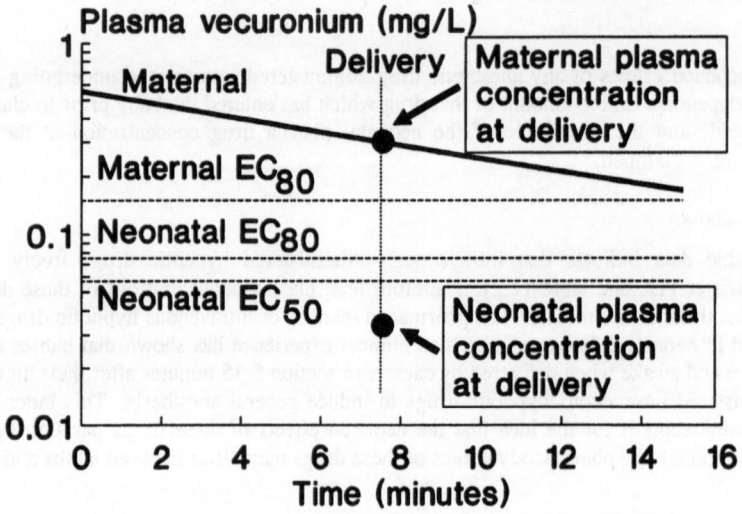

Figure 12.1: Maternal and fetal plasma concentrations of vecuronium after injection of a single dose of 0.05 mg/kg into the mother. Fetal plasma concentration is 0.11 that in the mother.

EXAMPLE 12.1.

Consider the administration of 0.05 mg/kg vecuronium to a woman undergoing caesarean section. Assume that the kinetic parameters of vecuronium in pregnant women are not significantly different from those in nonpregnant women. Let the time between injection to delivery be a very rapid 7.5 minutes. Will this dose of vecuronium have a significant effect on the neonate?

Vecuronium kinetic and dynamic data in adults

- MEC = EC_{80} = 0.15 mg/L.
- $t_{1/2\alpha}$ = 7.5 min.
- $t_{1/2\beta}$ = 53 min.
- A_x = 10.08 kg/L.
- B_x = 1.03 kg/L.

Maternal vecuronium plasma concentrations

- A = dose x A_x = 0.05 x 10.08 = 0.504 mg/L.

- $B = dose \times B_x = 0.05 \times 1.03 = 0.051$ mg/L.

- C_0 = initial plasma concentration = $A + B = 0.504 + 0.051 = 0.555$ mg/L.

- At time = 7.5 min = $1 \times t_{1/2\alpha}$, $n = 1$, and $N = 0.1415$.
  $C_t = A/2^n + B/2^N = 0.504/2 + 0.051/2^{0.1415} = 0.3$ mg/L, which is greater than the EC_{80} of vecuronium in adults. Therefore the mother is paralyzed at this time.

Neonatal plasma concentration at delivery

- F/M ratio of vecuronium at delivery = 0.11 [table 12.2].
- The maternal plasma vecuronium concentration at delivery = 0.3 mg/L. Therefore the neonatal plasma vecuronium concentration at delivery = $0.11 \times 0.3 = 0.033$ mg/L.

Consequences for the neonate

- For infants aged 2 months to one year, vecuronium $EC_{50} = 0.057$ mg/L, and $EC_{80} = 0.075$ mg/L [16].
- The neonatal plasma vecuronium concentration at delivery = 0.033 mg/L. This is a concentration which is well below the EC_{50}. Such a plasma vecuronium concentration will produce no clinically significant muscle relaxation in the neonate.

The same calculations can be made for other non-depolarizing muscle relaxant drugs.

REFERENCES

1. Lund CJ, Donovan JC: Blood volume during pregnancy. Significance of plasma and red cell volumes. *American Journal of Obstetrics & Gynecology*, 1967: 98: 393-403.
2. Lees MM, et al: A study of the cardiac output at rest throughout pregnancy. *Journal of Obstetrics and Gynaecology of the British Commonwealth*, 1967: 74: 319-328.
3. Hendricks CH: The hemodynamics of a uterine contraction. *American Journal of Obstetrics & Gynecology*, 1958: 76: 969-981.
4. Lees MM, et al: The circulatory effects of recumbent postural change in late pregnancy. *Clinical Science*, 1967: 32: 453-465.
5. Munnell EW, Taylor HC: Liver blood flow in pregnancy - hepatic vein catheterization. *Journal of Clinical Investigation*, 1947: 26: 952-956.
6. Altman PL, et al (editors), "Handbook of Circulation", published W.B. Saunders Co., U.S.A., 1959, Library of Congress Number 59-15183, pages 115-125.

7. Morgan DJ, et al: Pharmacokinetics and plasma binding of thiopental. II: Studies at cesarean section. *Anesthesiology*, 1981: 54: 474-480.
8. Morgan D, et al: Disposition of meperidine in pregnancy. *Clinical Pharmacology & Therapeutics*, 1978: 23: 288-295.
9. Kuhnert BR, et al: Meperidine disposition in mother, neonate, and nonpregnant females. *Clinical Pharmacology & Therapeutics*, 1980: 27: 486-491.
10. Duvaldestin P, et al: The placental transfer of pancuronium and its pharmacokinetics during caesarean section. *Acta Anaesthesiologica Scandinavica*, 1978: 22: 327-333.
11. Dailey PA, et al: Pharmacokinetics, placental transfer, and neonatal effects of vecuronium and pancuronium administered during cesarean section. *Anesthesiology*, 1984: 60: 569-574.
12. Hill MD, Abramson FP: The significance of plasma protein binding on the Fetal/Maternal distribution of drugs at steady state. *Clinical Pharmacokinetics*, 1988: 14: 156-170.
13. Crawford JS, Gardiner JE: Some aspects of obstetric anaesthesia. Part II. The use of relaxant drugs. *British Journal of Anaesthesia*, 1956: 28: 154-158.
14. Thomas J, et al: The placental transfer of alcuronium. *British Journal of Anaesthesia*, 1969: 41: 297-302.
15. Kanto J, Klotz U: Pharmacokinetic implications for the clinical use of atropine, scopolamine and glycopyrrolate. *Acta Anaesthesiologica Scandinavica*, 1988: 32: 69-78.
16. Fisher DM, et al: Vecuronium kinetics and dynamics in anesthetized infants and children. *Clinical Pharmacology & Therapeutics*, 1985: 37: 402-406.
17. Flynn PJ, et al: Use of atracurium in caesarean section. *British Journal of Anaesthesia*, 1984: 56: 599-605.

Chapter 13

Renal Failure

The kidneys play an important role in the elimination of many drugs used in anesthesia. They eliminate both unchanged drugs and their metabolites. Renal failure reduces the elimination of drugs and drug metabolites which are eliminated in the urine. In addition to this, renal failure also causes changes in body physiology which can also affect the pharmacology of anesthetic drugs.

PHYSIOLOGICAL AND KINETIC CHANGES

Some of the changes of physiology induced by renal failure, and their effects on drug pharmacokinetics will now be discussed.

Changes in extracellular fluid volume

The extracellular fluid volume of persons with renal failure is very variable. Extracellular fluid volume depends on whether the person has high, normal or low output renal failure, daily fluid intake and renal dialysis. A person with high output renal failure may actually be dehydrated, and so have an extracellular fluid volume which is lower than normal. Those with zero, or low output renal failure may be edematous due to fluid intake in excess of output. Extracellular fluid volume is increased in the latter situation.

Changes of extracellular fluid volume affect the distribution volumes of fat insoluble drugs, as these distribute mainly throughout the extracellular fluid volume.

Altered chemical composition of plasma and tissues

The chemical composition of all body fluids is altered by uremia. Plasma urea, uric acid and creatinine concentrations are increased. Hypocalcemia, hypermagnesemia and hyperkalemia may occur. Mild metabolic acidosis occurs frequently in patients with chronic renal failure. All these changes alter the chemical composition of blood and many other tissues. These changes of chemical environment can alter the interactions of drugs with the plasma proteins, receptors and tissues that bind them.

Table 13.1.

This table shows the percentage of an intravenously injected drug that is excreted unchanged in the urine in the first 24 hours in normal persons, and the effects of chronic renal failure on the kinetics of those drugs.

DRUG	% dose excreted unchanged in urine per 24 hours in normal persons	% Protein binding (change in renal failure)	$t_{1/2\beta}$ (change in renal failure)	V_d (change in renal failure)	Cl (change in renal failure)
Thiopental	minimal	↓[1,2]	0[1,2]	0	0
Propofol	<0.3[3]	?	0[4]	?	?
Morphine	10[5]	?	0[5,6]	0/↓	0
Fentanyl	6[7]	?	↓[8]	?	?
Alfentanil	<0.4[9]	↓[11]	0[10,11]	0/↑	0
Sufentanil	?	?	0[12]	0	0
Gallamine	>70[13]	?	↑[14]	↑	↓
Alcuronium	80[15]	?	↑[15]	?	?
Tubocurarine	40[16]	0[17]	↑[16]	?	?
Pancuronium	30[18]	?	↑[19]	↑	↓
Vecuronium	20[20]	?	↑[21]	0	↓
Atracurium	?	?	0[22]	0/↓	0
Pyridostigmine	>80[23]	?	↑[23]	0	↓
Neostigmine	67[24]	?	↑[24]	0	↓

↑ increased above value in normal healthy adult.
↓ decreased below value in normal healthy adult.
0 no change.
? unknown.

Changes in cardiac output

Many persons with severe chronic renal failure have a surgically constructed arteriovenous fistula for hemodialysis. This reduces peripheral vascular resistance to such a degree that cardiac output is significantly increased. As cardiopulmonary anatomy is unchanged by such a fistula, all the increased cardiac output passes through the pulmonary vessels and cardiac chambers.

This has possible consequences on pre-recirculation phase kinetics. For example, right-to-left heart circulation time is reduced, and so intravenously injected drugs will arrive in the aorta sooner than in persons without a shunt [see chapter 2]. Another theoretical effect is due to a reduction of the systemic vascular resistance as a result of the arteriovenous shunt. A reduction of the systemic vascular resistance increases left ventricular ejection fraction, and possibly the pre-recirculation phase peak concentrations too.

Reduced plasma protein concentration and drug binding

Chronic renal failure causes a reduction of plasma protein binding of anesthetic drugs in one or both of two ways. The chemical environment within the plasma is changed, and this may reduce the binding of drugs to plasma proteins. Persons with chronic renal failure have lower than normal plasma protein concentrations, which reduces the total amount of plasma protein able to bind drugs. Thiopental is an example of a drug whose plasma protein binding is reduced by both mechanisms during uremia [25]. The effects of reduced plasma protein drug binding have been discussed in chapter 8.

Reduced excretion of unchanged drug

The excretion, and so the clearances of drugs which are excreted to a significant degree as unchanged drug in the urine are reduced by renal failure. This particularly applies to the neuro-muscular blocking drugs [see table 13.1]. The elimination half lives of these drugs can be much prolonged in persons with renal failure. One exception to this rule is atracurium, whose elimination by means of the Hoffman reaction is independent of changes in renal function.

Anticholinesterase drugs also undergo predominantly renal excretion, and their half lives are fortunately also prolonged by renal failure [table 13.1]. An implication of this is that while renal failure may prolong the action of some muscle relaxants, it also prolongs the action of their antagonists, the anticholinesterases.

Table 13.2.

Anesthetic drugs known to have active metabolites which are excreted in the urine.

DRUG	Active metabolite	Activity relative to parent drug	Accumulation of metabolite occurs in renal failure?
Morphine [5]	morphine-glucuronide	less	yes
Meperidine [26]	norpethidine	less	yes
Phenoperidine [27]	meperidine, norpethidine	less	yes
Pancuronium [28]	3-hydroxypancuronium	less	yes

Reduced excretion of active drug metabolites

Some drugs have pharmacologically active metabolites whose main route of excretion is in the urine. Examples of such drugs are listed in table 13.2. A reduction of renal clearance of such metabolites may result in their accumulation after repeated administration, or administration of large doses of the parent drug.

EFFECTS OF RENAL FAILURE ON DRUG PHARMACODYNAMICS

The effects of anesthetic drugs appear to be unchanged by renal failure. This is shown by the lack of any change of the rapidity of onset, or dose-effect relationship of drugs such as thiopental [1], vecuronium [21,29], atracurium [30] and gallamine [31] in persons with renal failure. The above means that the dosages of anesthetic drugs need not be different to those required for normal persons.

However, renal failure can change drug dynamics if it also causes hypoproteinemia. Hypoproteinaemia decreases plasma protein drug binding, which results in increased tissue drug concentrations. For example, the dose of thiopental required to induce hypnosis is normal in normoproteinemic [1], but reduced below normal in hypoproteinemic persons with renal failure [2]. This is expected as reduced percentage protein binding increases brain and tissue thiopental concentrations above normal [25].

CLINICAL CONSEQUENCES

The clinical consequences of these changes vary somewhat with the drug group under consideration.

Induction agents

This has already been discussed in the section on the pharmacodynamic changes induced by renal failure.

Opiates

Renal failure does reduce the protein binding of alfentanil [11], and may also affect the protein binding of other opiates. However the kinetics of opiates such as morphine, fentanyl, alfentanil and sufentanil are not significantly altered in persons with renal failure [table 13.1]. Clinical experience also shows that the dynamics of opiates are unlikely to be significantly changed by renal failure, as doses and requirement of these drugs during anesthesia are the same as in healthy persons.

Muscle relaxants

The predominant route of elimination of d-tubocurarine, alcuronium and gallamine is by excretion of the unchanged drug in the urine. Other non-depolarizing muscle relaxants also undergo significant elimination in the urine as the unchanged drug. So it is only to be expected that renal failure significantly changes the elimination kinetics of these drugs. This change is usually expressed as reduced clearance of non-depolarizing muscle relaxants. The only exception to this rule is atracurium which is rapidly eliminated in blood by the Hoffman reaction [28].

Reduced renal clearances of non-depolarizing muscle relaxants means that the effect of normal doses of these drugs may be significantly prolonged by renal failure. This is shown in example 13.1 for gallamine, a drug which is exclusively excreted unchanged in the urine.

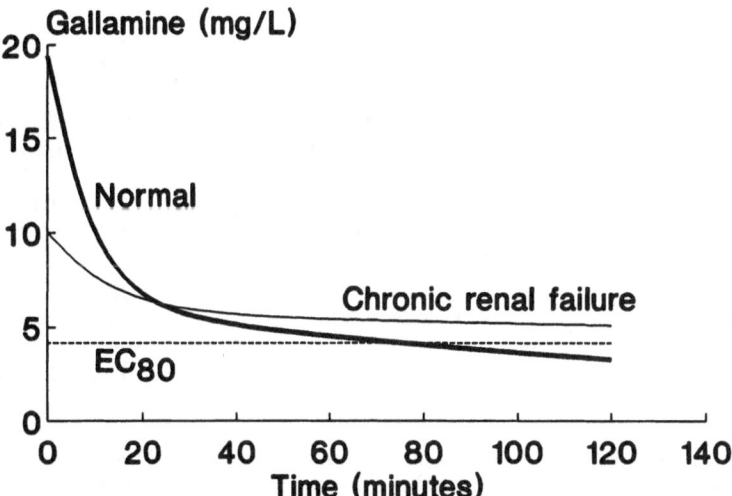

Figure 13.1: Plasma concentration-time curves of gallamine 1.5 mg/kg administered to a person with renal failure and one with normal renal function. A dose of 1.5 mg/kg is a very normal clinical dose for this drug. Elimination and duration of effect are both prolonged by renal failure [see example 13.1].

EXAMPLE 13.1:

Consider the change of plasma gallamine concentration with time in relation to the EC_{80} of intravenous bolus doses of 1.5 mg/kg gallamine administered to a patient with renal failure, and one with normal renal function.

This is quite a normal dose of gallamine. Use data on gallamine kinetics in healthy adults, and adults with renal failure from Ramzan et al (1981) [14].

	Normal	Renal failure
Dose (mg/kg)	1.5	1.5
EC_{80} = MEC (mg/L)	4.17	4.17
$t_{1/2\alpha}$ (minutes)	5.65	8.88
$t_{1/2\beta}$ (minutes)	131	752
V_1 (L/kg)	0.1	0.15
V_β (L/kg)	0.23	0.29
Cl (L/h/kg)	0.072	0.0144
A_x (kg/L)	5.84	2.86
B_x (kg/L)	4.16	3.81
A = dose x A_x (mg/L)	8.76	4.29
B = dose x B_x (mg/L)	6.24	5.72

Time (min)	n	N	Concn. (mg/L)	n	N	Concn. (mg/L)
At 0 x $t_{1/2\alpha}$	0	0	15	0	0	10.05
At 1 x $t_{1/2\alpha}$	1	0.043	10.44	1	0.012	7.81
At 2 x $t_{1/2\alpha}$	2	0.086	8.07	2	0.024	6.69
At 3 x $t_{1/2\alpha}$	3	0.129	6.8	3	0.035	6.11
At 4 x $t_{1/2\alpha}$	4	0.173	6.08	4	0.047	5.8
At 1 x $t_{1/2\beta}$	23.18	1	3.12 < MEC	84.68	1	2.86 < MEC

The results of these calculations show a number of very interesting features. The initial plasma gallamine concentration is not as high in the renal failure patient as in the normal patient. So the maximum muscle relaxant effect due to such a dose is likely to be less, and rate of onset of effect slower in the renal failure patient. Another feature is that the termination of useful drug effect, (defined as a plasma drug concentration which drops below the EC_{80}), is by elimination in both patients. However, the elimination half life is much longer in the renal failure patient than in the normal patient, and so the effect also lasts longer [see figure 13.1].

There is a belief among some anesthesiologists that the muscle paralysis due to non-depolarizing muscle relaxants such as alcuronium, d-tubocurarine, and especially gallamine is always prolonged in persons with renal failure. This is incorrect. The prolonged duration of muscle relaxation due to these drugs is a dose related phenomenon. Renal failure does not change the concentration-effect curves of the non-depolarizing muscle relaxants [21,29,30,31]. However the kinetics of these drugs are changed such that lower REPEAT, but not INITIAL doses are required.

It is possible to select a dose of a muscle relaxant such that the effect is terminated only by (re)distribution and not elimination [see also example 5.9]. This makes it possible to use drugs such as gallamine and alcuronium safely in persons with renal failure, especially when one considers that the elimination half lives of their antagonists, the anti-cholinesterases, are also lengthened by renal failure.

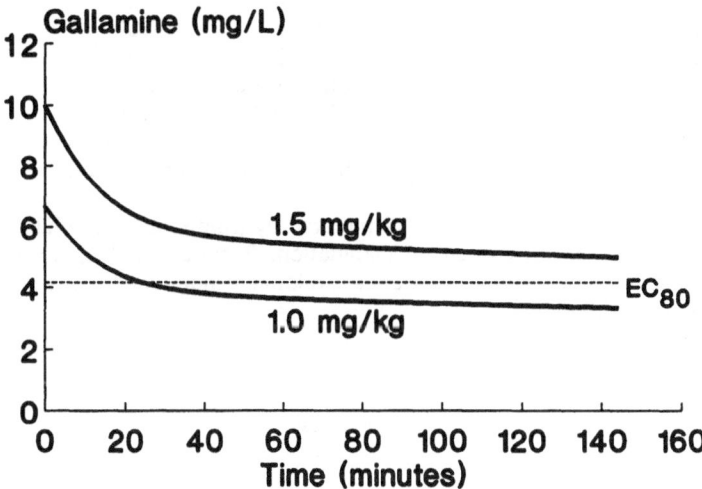

Figure 13.2: Plasma concentration-time curves of a 1 mg/kg and 1.5 mg/kg doses of gallamine administered to persons with renal failure. These curves are shown in relation to the EC_{80}. It is evident that the effect of the 1 mg/kg dose is terminated by (re)distribution, while that of the 1.5 mg/kg dose is terminated by elimination [see example 13.2].

EXAMPLE 13.2:

Consider the plasma concentration-time curves of gallamine in relation to its EC_{80} after administration of two different bolus doses to a person with renal failure. The doses are 1.0 and 1.5 mg/kg, and kinetic parameters are from Ramzan et al (1981) [14].

$MEC = EC_{80}$ (mg/L)	4.17
$t_{1/2\alpha}$ (minutes)	8.88
$t_{1/2\beta}$ (minutes)	752

		1.0 mg/kg	1.5 mg/kg
A_x (kg/L)		2.86	
B_x (kg/L)		3.81	
Dose		**1.0 mg/kg**	**1.5 mg/kg**
$A = dose \times A_x$ (mg/L)		2.86	4.29
$B = dose \times B_x$ (mg/L)		3.81	5.72

Time (min)	n	N	Concn. (mg/L)	Concn. (mg/L)
At 0 x $t_{1/2\alpha}$	0	0	6.67	10
At 1 x $t_{1/2\alpha}$	1	0.012	5.21	7.81
At 2 x $t_{1/2\alpha}$	2	0.024	4.46	6.69
At 3 x $t_{1/2\alpha}$	3	0.035	4.08 < MEC	6.11
At 4 x $t_{1/2\alpha}$	4	0.047	3.87 < MEC	5.8
At 1 x $t_{1/2\beta}$	84.68	1	1.91 < MEC	2.86 < MEC

The effect of the lower dose is terminated by (re)distribution while that of the higher dose is terminated by elimination. Because of this, duration of muscle relaxation due to the lower dose is relatively independent of the degree of renal dysfunction.

REFERENCES

1. Christensen JH, et al: Pharmacokinetics and pharmacodynamics of thiopental in patients undergoing renal transplantation. *Acta Anaesthesiologica Scandinavica*, 1983: 27: 513-518.
2. Burch PG, Stanski DR: Decreased protein binding and thiopental kinetics. *Clinical Pharmacology & Therapeutics*, 1982: 32: 212-217.
3. Cockshott ID: Propofol ("Diprivan") pharmacokinetics and metabolism - an overview. *Postgraduate Medical Journal*, 1985: 61 (suppl. 3): 45-50.
4. Morcos WE, Payne JP: The induction of anaesthesia with propofol ("Diprivan") compared in normal and renal failure patients. *Postgraduate Medical Journal*, 1985: 61 (suppl. 3): 62-63.
5. Chauvin M, et al: Morphine pharmacokinetics in renal failure. *Anesthesiology*, 1987: 66: 327-331.
6. Aitkenhead AR, et al: Pharmacokinetics of single-dose i.v. morphine in normal volunteers and patients with end-stage renal failure. *British Journal of Anaesthesia*, 1984: 56: 813-819.
7. McClain DA, Hug CC: Intravenous fentanyl kinetics. *Clinical Pharmacology & Therapeutics*, 1980: 28: 106-114.
8. Corall IM, et al: Plasma concentrations of fentanyl in normal surgical patients and those with severe renal and hepatic disease. *British Journal of Anaesthesia*, 1980: 52: 101P.
9. Schuttler J, Stoekel H: Alfentanil (R 39209) ein neues kurzwirkendes Opioid. *Der Anaesthesist*, 1982: 31: 10-14.
10. Sear JW, et al: Disposition of alfentanil in patients with chronic renal failure. *British Journal of Anaesthesia*, 1986: 58: 812P.

11. Chauvin M, et al: Pharmacokinetics of alfentanil in chronic renal failure. *Anesthesia and Analgesia*, 1987: 66: 53-56.
12. Davis PJ, et al: Pharmacokinetics of sufentanil in adolescent patients with chronic renal failure. *Anesthesia and Analgesia*, 1988: 67: 268-271.
13. Agoston S, et al: A preliminary investigation of the renal and hepatic excretion of gallamine triethiodide in man. *British Journal of Anaesthesia*, 1978: 50: 345-351.
14. Ramzan MI, et al: Gallamine disposition in surgical patients with chronic renal failure. *British Journal of Clinical Pharmacology*, 1981: 12: 141-147.
15. Raaflaub J, Frey P: Zur Pharmackokinetik von Diallyl-nor-toxiferin beim Menschen. *Arzneimittelforschung*, 1972: 22: 73-78.
16. Miller RD, et al: The pharmacokinetics of d-tubocurarine in man with and without renal failure. *Journal of Pharmacology and Experimental Therapeutics*, 1977: 202: 1-7.
17. Ghoneim MM, et al: Binding of d-tubocurarine to plasma proteins in normal man and in patients with hepatic or renal disease. *Anesthesiology*, 1973: 39: 410-415.
18. Agoston S, et al: The fate of pancuronium bromide in man. *Acta Anaesthesiologica Scandinavica*, 1973: 17: 267-275.
19. McLeod K, et al: Pharmacokinetics of pancuronium in patients with normal and impaired renal function. *British Journal of Anaesthesia*, 1976: 48: 341-345.
20. Bencini A, "Clinical pharmacokinetics of vecuronium bromide", pages 25-37, in "Clinical Experiences with Norcuron", ed. Agoston S, Excerpta Current Clinical Practice Series 6, pub. 1982, ISBN 90-219-9610-3.
21. Lynam DP, et al: The pharmacodynamics and pharmacokinetics of vecuronium in patients anesthetized with isoflurane with normal renal function or with renal failure. *Anesthesiology*, 1988: 69: 227-231.
22. Ward S, Neill EAM: Pharmacokinetics of atracurium in acute hepatic failure (with acute renal failure). *British Journal of Anaesthesia*, 1983: 55: 1169-1172.
23. Cronnelly R, et al: Pyridostigmine kinetics with and without renal function. *Clinical Pharmacology & Therapeutics*, 1980: 28: 78-81.
24. Cronnelly R, et al: Renal function and the pharmacokinetics neostigmine in anesthetized man. *Anesthesiology*, 1979: 51: 222-226.
25. Ghoneim MM, et al: Binding of thiopental to plasma proteins: Effects on distribution in the brain and heart. *Anesthesiology*, 1978: 45: 635-639.
26. Mather LE, Meffin PJ: Clinical pharmacokinetics pethidine. *Clinical Pharmacokinetics*, 1978: 3: 352-368.
27. Isherwood CN, et al: Elimination of phenoperidine in liver disease. *British Journal of Anaesthesia*, 1984: 56: 843-847.
28. Hilgenberg JC: Comparison of the pharmacology of vecuronium and atracurium with that of other currently available muscle relaxants. *Anesthesia and Analgesia*, 1983: 62: 524-531.
29. Fahey MR, et al: Pharmacokinetics of ORG NC45 (Norcuron) in patients with and without renal failure. *British Journal of Anaesthesia*, 1981: 53: 1049-1053.
30. Fahey MR, et al: Pharmacokinetics and pharmacodynamics of atracurium in normal and renal failure patients. *Anesthesiology*, 1983: 59: A263.
31. Ramzan MI, et al: Gallamine disposition in surgical patients with chronic renal failure. *British Journal of Clinical Pharmacology*, 1981: 12: 141-147.

Chapter 14

Hepatic Dysfunction

The liver is the metabolic powerhouse of the body. Hepatic blood flow is 28% of the cardiac output. It produces nearly all the plasma proteins, and is responsible for the metabolism of most drugs. So hepatic disease can produce extensive changes in body physiology, and these may alter the pharmacology of anesthetic drugs.

PHYSIOLOGICAL AND KINETIC CHANGES

Some of the changes induced by hepatic disease are discussed below, together with their effects on drug kinetics.

Increased cardiac output

Cardiac output is elevated above normal levels in all persons with hepatic dysfunction, regardless of whether the cause is hepatocellular or cholestatic. The cause of this is a reduction of the systemic vascular resistance together with a baroreflex mediated elevation of cardiac output, despite a reduction of myocardial contractility due to hyperbilirubinemia.

Increased cardiac output means that the circulation times between most points of the body are decreased [see chapter 2]. So the time to onset of drug action after intravenous bolus injection of many drugs may be reduced in patients with hepatic dysfunction.

Reduced plasma protein concentrations

Hepatic production of many plasma proteins, including albumin, is reduced by hepatic dysfunction. This can cause peripheral edema, in addition to which the amount of albumin available for drug binding is reduced.

Bilirubin binds to the same sites on albumin molecules as many drugs. So hyperbilirubinemia reduces the number of available drug binding sites on albumin by competing with drugs for the same binding sites.

Table 14.1.
Effect of chronic hepatic disease (HD) on protein binding and elimination kinetics of various intravenous anesthetic drugs.

DRUG	% dose metabolized or excreted unchanged in bile per 24 hrs (normal)	% Protein binding (change in HD)	$t_{1/2\beta}$ (change in HD)	V_d (change in HD)	Cl (change in HD)
Thiopental	most	↓[1]	0[1]	0	0
Hexobarbital	most	?	0[2]	0	0
Etomidate	most	↓[3]	↑[4]	↑	0
Morphine	most	↓[5]	↑[5]	0	↓
Meperidine	most	?	↑[6]	0	↓
Pentazocine	most	?	↑[6]	0	↓
Phenoperidine	?	?	↑[4]	0	↓
Fentanyl	most	?	0[7]	0	0
Alfentanil	most	?	↑[8]	0	↓
Sufentanil	?	0[9]	0[9]	0	0
Gallamine	0	?	0[10]	↑	0
Pancuronium	30	?	↑[11]	↑	↓
Vecuronium	most	?	↑[12]	0	↓
Atracurium	0	?	0[13]	0	0

↑ increased above value in healthy adult.
↓ decreased below value in healthy adult.
0 no change.
? unknown.

Increased extracellular fluid volume

Some persons with hepatic dysfunction may have ascites and/or peripheral edema. Both increase the extracellular fluid volume. Peripheral edema is a result of renal water retention and hypoproteinemia. Ascites can be be caused by increased portal venous pressure, obstruction of hepatic lymph drainage, as well as renal water retention and hypoproteinemia. The effect of both ascites and peripheral edema is to increase the volumes of distribution of fat insoluble drugs.

Reduced metabolic function

Many drugs used in anesthesia undergo a greater or lesser degree of hepatic metabolism. The rates of metabolism, and hence clearances of such drugs are reduced by hepatic dysfunction.

Reduced drug clearance

Drug clearance is a function of both the elimination of the unchanged drug as well as metabolism. Most anaesthetic drugs are metabolized to some degree in the liver, and some are also excreted to a significant degree in bile as unchanged drug. The effect of severe liver dysfunction is to reduce hepatic drug clearance, which in turn causes the elimination half lives of the affected drugs to be lengthened [see table 14.1].

Increased central compartment and distribution volume

The central compartment and distribution volumes of some drugs are increased by severe chronic liver disease [see table 14.1]. This may be the result of ascites and edema increasing the pharmacokinetic compartmental volumes of very water soluble drugs which distribute mainly in the extracellular fluid volume, or it may be due to reduced protein binding. In either case, if the clearance of the drug is either unchanged or reduced, the elimination half life is lengthened [see equation 3.28].

CLINICAL CONSEQUENCES

The clinical consequences of severe hepatic disease for the administration of intravenous anesthetic drugs differ according to the type of drug.

Induction agents

Hypnotic doses of intravenous hypnotic drugs such as thiopental [1] are unchanged in patients with hepatic cirrhosis. However a reduced level of consciousness due to the presence of hepatic encephalopathy may reduce the hypnotic dose required.

The reduced degree of plasma protein binding may exacerbate the cardiovascular depression caused by an induction dose of these drugs [see chapter 8].

Elimination half lives of anesthetic induction agents are increased in persons with hepatic dysfunction. However this is of little clinical significance when these drugs are administered as an intravenous bolus. In this situation the termination of hypnosis is by (re)distribution, and not elimination. If an induction agent is administered as an intravenous infusion to maintain hypnosis/sedation, the infusion rate required may be lower than usual because of reduced drug clearance.

Opiates

Table 14.1 clearly shows that the plasma protein binding and clearance of the opiates are reduced, and the elimination half lives are increased in persons with severe hepatic disease. The reduction of plasma protein binding of some opiates such as morphine [see table 14.1] implies that the clinical effect of a given dose of some opiates may be enhanced due to the increased free fraction the drug at any given concentration, and indeed this is thought to occur with meperidine [6].

Non-depolarizing muscle relaxants

The effects of severe hepatic disease have not been studied as extensively for the neuromuscular blocking drugs. Both the kinetics and dynamics of gallamine [10] and atracurium [13] are relatively unaffected. These drugs can be administered as usual to persons with hepatic dysfunction.

The kinetics of drugs such as vecuronium and pancuronium are altered by hepatic disease. Their elimination half lives are prolonged due to either increased distribution volume, reduced clearance or both [see table 14.1]. The concentration-effect curves of these drugs are unchanged from those in healthy persons [12]. However the dose of relaxant required to achieve a given plasma concentration and effect is increased because of increased central compartment and distribution volumes induced by hepatic dysfunction, e.g. as for pancuronium [11]. This means that the effect of a given dose is less than expected in a healthy person, and the clinician speaks of "resistance" to the effects of the drug [see example 14.1].

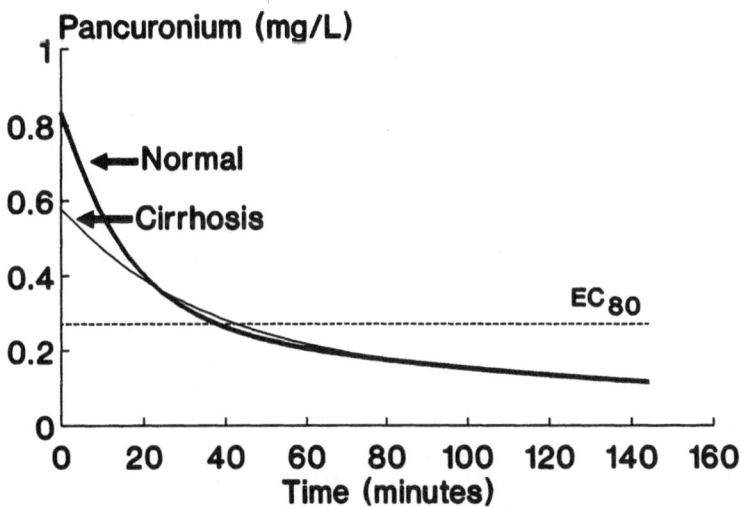

Figure 14.1: Pancuronium plasma concentration-time curves in normal and cirrhotic persons after administration of a 0.1 mg/kg intravenous bolus dose. The curves are shown in relation to the EC_{80}. See example 14.1 for more detailed information about this figure.

EXAMPLE 14.1:

Consider the administration of an intravenous bolus dose of 0.1 mg/kg pancuronium to a person with hepatic dysfunction, and to another person who is healthy. Use the methods outlined in chapter 5, and the kinetic data of Duvaldestin et al (1978) [11] for patients with chronic hepatic cirrhosis.

	Normal	Cirrhosis
Dose (mg/kg)	0.1	0.1
EC_{80} (mg/L)	0.27	0.27
$t_{1/2\alpha}$ (minutes)	10.7	23.7
$t_{1/2\beta}$ (minutes)	114	208
V_1 (L/kg)	0.12	0.173
V_β (L/kg)	0.279	0.416
Cl (L/h/kg)	0.11	0.087
A_x (kg/L)	5.54	3.93
B_x (kg/L)	2.8	1.85
A = dose x A_x (mg/L)	0.554	0.393
B = dose x B_x (mg/L)	0.28	0.185

Time (min)	n	N	Concn. (mg/L)	n	N	Concn. (mg/L)
At 0 x $t_{1/2\alpha}$	0	0	0.834	0	0	0.578
At 1 x $t_{1/2\alpha}$	1	0.094	0.54	1	0.114	0.367
At 2 x $t_{1/2\alpha}$	2	0.188	0.384	2	0.228	0.256 < MEC
At 3 x $t_{1/2\alpha}$	3	0.28	0.3	3	0.342	0.195 < MEC
At 4 x $t_{1/2\alpha}$	4	0.375	0.25 < MEC	4	0.456	0.159 < MEC
At 1 x $t_{1/2\beta}$	10.65	1	0.14 < MEC	8.77	1	0.093 < MEC

The calculations above and figure 14.1 show that the peak plasma pancuronium concentration is significantly lower in persons with hepatic cirrhosis than in normal persons. This means that the initial degree of muscle relaxation due to a given dose of pancuronium is less in cirrhotic than in normal persons. Such a phenomenon gives rise to the impression that persons with hepatic dysfunction are "resistant" to pancuronium. In addition to this, pancuronium clearance is reduced by hepatic dysfunction, and so accumulation may occur when repeat doses are not administered in response to clinical requirements.

REFERENCES

1.   Pandele G, et al: Thiopental pharmacokinetics in patients with cirrhosis. *Anesthesiology*, 1983: 59: 123-126.
2.   Richter E, et al: Disposition of hexobarbital in intra- and extrahepatic cholestasis in man and the influence of drug metabolism-inducing agents. *European Journal of Clinical Pharmacology*, 1980: 17: 197-202.
3.   Carlos R, et al: Plasma protein binding of etomidate in in patients with renal failure or hepatic cirrhosis. *Clinical Pharmacokinetics*, 1979: 4: 144-148.
4.   Sear JW: General kinetic and dynamic principles and their application to continuous infusion anaesthesia. *Anaesthesia*, 1983: supplement, vol 38: 10-25.
5.   Mazoit J-X, et al: Pharmacokinetics of unchanged morphine normal and cirrhotic subjects. *Anesthesia and Analgesia*, 1987: 66: 293-298.
6.   Neal EA, et al: Enhanced bioavailability and decreased clearance of analgesics in patients with cirrhosis. *Gastroenterology*, 1979: 77: 96-102.
7.   Haberer JP, et al: Fentanyl pharmacokinetics in anaesthetized patients with cirrhosis. *British Journal of Anaesthesia*, 1982: 54: 1267-1269.
8.   Levron JC, et al,(1983), Pharmacokinetics of alfentanil in surgical patients with normal and disturbed liver function. Unpublished data, on file Janssen Pharmaceutica.
9.   Chauvin M, et al: Sufentanil pharmacokinetics in patients with cirrhosis. *Anesthesiology*, 1988: 69: A458.
10. Ramzan IM, et al: Pharmacokinetics and pharmacodynamics of gallamine triethiodide in patients with total biliary obstruction. *Anesthesia and Analgesia*, 1981: 60: 289-296.
11. Duvaldestin P, et al: Pancuronium pharmacokinetics in patients with liver cirrhosis. *British Journal of Anaesthesia*, 1978: 50: 1131-1135.
12. Lebrault C, et al: Pharmacokinetics and pharmacodynamics of vecuronium in patients with cholestasis. *British Journal of Anaesthesia*, 1986: 58, 93.
13. Ward S, Neill EAM: Pharmacokinetics of atracurium in acute hepatic failure (with acute renal failure). *British Journal of Anaesthesia*, 1983: 55: 1169-1172.

Appendix - A

Kinetic and Dynamic Parameters

This appendix contains a table of the pharmacokinetic and pharmacodynamic variables of many drugs used in intravenous anesthesia. The prime purpose of this table is to present those variables which are of most use in performing clinical kinetic and dynamic calculations. Therefore only a few kinetic and dynamic variables are listed for each drug, and certainly no physico-chemical data. These latter are presented in appendix-B.

Choice of kinetic model

The data listed in this table are for 2-compartment pharmacokinetic model. This model provides a reasonably good description of anesthetic drug kinetics after intravenous bolus injection and during infusions.

Pharmacokinetic variables

The derivation and meanings of pharmacokinetic variables such as A_x, B_x, $t_{1/2\alpha}$, α, $t_{1/2\beta}$, β, V_c, V_β and Cl have been explained extensively in chapter 3.

Readers should note that the table in this appendix lists clearance with the units L/h/kg instead of the more usual ml/min/kg. This is done in order to simplify calculation of drug infusion rates.

$t_{1/2}k_{eo}$

This is the concentration equilibration half life of drug exchange between plasma and the effect compartment [see chapter 4 for discussion].

MEC (Minimum Effective Concentration)

The MEC is the Minimum mean Effective plasma Concentration of a drug which is just sufficient to induce a given pharmacological effect [see chapter 4 for a more extensive discussion]. A plasma concentration of a drug equal to the MEC for a given effect due to that drug means that that effect is present in ONLY 50% of the persons participating in the studies cited. Drug concentrations which are 2-3 times the MEC are required to produce that same effect in more than 90% of persons.

MEC for hypnosis

This is the MEC for hypnosis for various hypnotic drugs. NOTE that the plasma concentration of a drug which is required to induce hypnosis alone is LESS than the concentrations required to induce hypnosis with loss of the eyelid, corneal, or pain reflexes. This is shown in tables 4.3 and 5.1.

MEC for EC_{80}

Non-depolarizing muscle relaxant effect is usually quantified by measuring the contraction force of an adductor pollicis longus muscle in response to supramaximal electrical stimulation of the ulnar nerve innervating it. Intra-abdominal surgery is just possible during relaxant/opiate/nitrous oxide/oxygen anesthesia if the contractile force of this muscle in response to a SINGLE stimulus is 80% less than the force measured without relaxants [47]. This force is equivalent to the degree of muscle relaxation present when a third twitch is just detectable in response to a "train-of-four" stimulus [48]. The steady state plasma concentration of a muscle relaxant drug capable of inducing such a degree of muscle paralysis is called the Effective Concentration at which 80% twitch height depression occurs. This is abbreviated to EC_{80}. Because of inter-personal variation, the EC_{80} is an average concentration for a given population. The EC_{80} is also the MEC for muscle relaxant drugs for a degree of muscle relaxation just sufficient to permit intra-abdominal surgery.

Aside from the fact that the EC_{80} is the MEC for muscle relaxants required for intra-abdominal surgery, there is another reason why the EC_{80} is such a useful MEC. Antagonism of non-depolarizing muscle relaxant drugs with anticholinesterases is usually complete within 10 minutes at this degree of muscle relaxation. Reversal of muscle paralysis takes significantly longer at greater degrees of muscle paralysis [45,46].

MEC for postoperative analgesia

This is the MEC of analgesic drugs at which effective POSTOPERATIVE analgesia occurs in AWAKE AND SPONTANEOUSLY BREATHING PATIENTS. The MEC for postoperative analgesia is NOT necessarily a plasma concentration of these analgesic drugs which is sufficient to suppress autonomic responses to surgical procedures or tracheal intubation. Plasma drug concentrations required to block responses to surgical stimuli and tracheal intubation are usually much higher. Such high drug concentrations of opioid drugs are often associated with significant respiratory depression or apnea.

MEC for tachycardia

This is the MEC of anticholinergic drugs which is capable of inducing a tachycardia.

INDUCTION AGENTS

DRUG	$t_{1/2\alpha}$ (min)	α (min^{-1})	$t_{1/2\beta}$ (min)	β (min^{-1})	V_c (L/kg)	V_β (L/kg)	Cl (L/h/kg)	A_x (kg/L)	B_x (kg/L)	MEC (hypnosis) (mg/L)	$t_{1/2}k_{eo}$ (min)
Thiopental	3.3[60]	0.21	781	0.0009	0.128	3.5	0.19	7.68	0.26	10[2]	1.2[50]
Methohexital	5.6[1]	0.124	234	0.003	0.35	3.7	0.65	2.65	0.21	3.4[3]	
Hexobarbital	23.4[4]	0.03	299	0.0023	0.54	1.4	0.2	1.25	0.6	10[4]	
Ketamine	11[5]	0.063	151	0.0046	0.86	4	1.1	0.98	0.18	1[6]	
Etomidate	2.6[7]	0.267	67	0.0103	0.3	2.2	1.39	3	0.33	0.21[8]	1.6[51]
Propofol	2.5[9]	0.277	55	0.013	0.63	4.7	3.55	1.44	0.15	1[10]	2.9[52]
Midazolam	18.6[11]	0.0373	164	0.0042	0.58	1.9	0.48	1.35	0.38	0.2[12]	5.4[53]
Diazepam	37.8[58]	0.0183	1746	0.0004	0.214	1.26	0.03	3.96	0.71	0.96[59]	1.63[53]
Alfentanil	3.8[31]	0.182	67	0.01	0.17	0.54	0.33	4.24	1.64	1.2[33]	1.1[54]

ANTICHOLINERGICS

DRUG	$t_{1/2\alpha}$ (min)	α (min^{-1})	$t_{1/2\beta}$ (min)	β (min^{-1})	V_c (L/kg)	$-V_\beta$ (L/kg)	Cl (L/h/kg)	A_x (kg/L)	B_x (kg/L)	MEC (tachycardia) (mg/L)	$t_{1/2}k_{eo}$ (min)
Atropine	1.7[41]	0.41	180	0.0038	0.09	1.6	0.41	10.65	0.46	0.03[42]	
Scopolamine	5.4[41]	0.128	114	0.0061	0.2	1.1	0.86	4.8	0.2	0.03[42]	

ANTICHOLINESTERASES

DRUG	$t_{1/2\alpha}$ (min)	α (min^{-1})	$t_{1/2\beta}$ (min)	β (min^{-1})	V_c (L/kg)	V_β (L/kg)	Cl (L/h/kg)	A_x (kg/L)	B_x (kg/L)	MEC (mg/L)	$t_{1/2}k_{eo}$ (min)
Neostigmine	3.4[43]	0.204	77	0.009	0.22	1.02	0.55	3.74	0.81	?	
Edrophonium	7.2[43]	0.096	110	0.0063	0.32	1.53	0.58	2.64	0.49	?	
Pyridostigmine	6.8[44]	0.102	112	0.0062	0.3	1.4	0.52	2.79	0.54	?	

MUSCLE RELAXANTS

DRUG	$t_{1/2\alpha}$ (min)	α (min^{-1})	$t_{1/2\beta}$ (min)	β (min^{-1})	V_c (L/kg)	V_β (L/kg)	Cl (L/h/kg)	A_x (kg/L)	B_x (kg/L)	MEC (EC$_{80}$) (mg/L)	$t_{1/2}k_{eo}$ (min)
Gallamine	6.7[13]	0.103	144	0.0048	0.1	0.23	0.065	5.83	4.17	7.2[14]	
Tubocurarine	6.2[15]	0.112	119	0.0058	0.1	0.39	0.135	7.82	2.18	0.63[14]	4.7[15]
Alcuronium	13.8[16]	0.05	199	0.0035	0.13	0.4	0.083	5.55	2.14	0.66[14]	
Pancuronium	10.7[17]	0.065	114	0.0061	0.12	0.3	0.11	5.54	2.8	0.27[14]	3.3[55]
Vecuronium	7.5[18]	0.092	53	0.013	0.09	0.4	0.32	10.08	1.03	0.15[14]	3.7[56]
Atracurium	2[19]	0.347	21	0.033	0.04	0.16	0.32	21	4.21	0.9[14]	5.9[62]

OPIATES

DRUG	$t_{1/2\alpha}$ (min)	α (min⁻¹)	$t_{1/2\beta}$ (min)	β (min⁻¹)	V_c (L/kg)	V_β (L/kg)	Cl (L/h/kg)	A_x (kg/L)	B_x (kg/L)	MEC (postop-analgesia) (mg/L)	$t_{1/2}k_{eo}$ (min)
Morphine	4.4[20]	0.158	111	0.0062	1.01	5.4	2.01	0.84	0.15	0.015[21]	
Methadone	6.1[22]	0.114	2100	0.0003	1.1	8.2	0.016	0.079	0.12	0.03[21,22]	
Meperidine	4.1[23]	0.169	192	0.0036	0.63	3.3	0.72	1.31	0.27	0.46[24]	
Pentazocine	?[25]	?	204	0.0034	?	5.6	1.2	?	?	0.1[26]	
Buprenorphine	2.1[61]	0.33	140	0.005	0.132	2.69	0.8	7.31	0.26	0.001[61]	
Phenoperidine	2.2[27]	0.315	193	0.0036	0.9	6.13	1.32	0.96	0.15	0.005[28]	
Fentanyl	9[29]	0.077	263	0.0026	0.77	3.81	0.65	1.09	0.21	0.001[30]	6.4[57]
Alfentanil	3.8[31]	0.182	67	0.01	0.17	0.54	0.33	4.24	1.64	0.1[32,49]	1.1[54]
Sufentanil	1.4[34]	0.495	164	0.0042	0.16	2.9	0.76	5.96	0.29	?	5.8[57]

ANTAGONISTS & ANALEPTICS

DRUG	$t_{1/2\alpha}$ (min)	α (min⁻¹)	$t_{1/2\beta}$ (min)	β (min⁻¹)	V_c (L/kg)	V_β (L/kg)	Cl (L/h/kg)	A_x (kg/L)	B_x (kg/L)	MEC (mg/L)	$t_{1/2}k_{eo}$ (min)
Naloxone	1.8[35]	0.385	19	0.036	0.81	2.4	5.3	0.91	0.32	?	
Doxapram	5.3[36]	0.1263	54	0.002	0.44	3.2	0.36	1.98	0.3	2-3[37]	
Physostigmine	2.3[38]	0.301	22	0.032	?	0.6	1.2	?	?	0.004[38]	
Flumazanil	?[39]	?	58	0.012	?	0.82	0.6	?	?	0.02[40]	

REFERENCES

1. Hudson RJ, et al: Pharmacokinetics of methohexital and thiopental in surgical patients. *Anesthesiology*, 1983: 59: 215-219.
2. Hudson RJ, et al: A model for studying depth of anesthesia and acute tolerance to thiopental. *Anesthesiology*, 1983: 59: 301-308.
3. Lauven PM, et al: Venous threshold concentrations of methohexitone. *Anesthesiology*, 1985: 63: A368.
4. Richter E, et al: Disposition of hexobarbital in intra- and extrahepatic cholestasis in man and the influence of drug metabolism-inducing agents. *European Journal of Clinical Pharmacology*, 1980: 17: 197-202.
5. Wieber J, et al: Pharmacokinetics of ketamine in man. *Der Anaesthesist*, 1975: 24: 260-263.
6. White PF, et al: Comparative pharmacology of the ketamine isomers. Studies in volunteers. *British Journal of Anaesthesia*, 1985: 57: 197-203.
7. Schüttler J, et al: Pharmakokinetische Untersuchungen uber Etomidat beim Menschen. *Der Anaesthesist*, 1980: 29: 658-661.
8. Schüttler J, et al: Infusion strategies to investigate the pharmacokinetics and pharmacodynamics of hypnotic drugs: etomidate as an example. *European Journal of Anaesthesiology*, 1985: 2: 133-142.
9. Adam HK, et al: Pharmacokinetic evaluation of ICI 35868 in man. *British Journal of Anaesthesia*, 1983: 55: 97-102.
10. Shafer A, et al: Pharmacokinetics and pharmacodynamics of propofol infusion. *Anesthesiology*, 1987: 67: A668.
11. Greenblatt DJ, et al: Effect of age, gender, and obesity on midazolam kinetics. *Anesthesiology*, 1984: 61: 27-35.
12. Personal communication Professor Dr. P.J. Hennis, Head of Department of Anesthesiology, University Hospital Groningen, Groningen, the Netherlands.
13. Ramzan MI, et al: Pharmacokinetic studies in man with gallamine triethiodide. I. Single and multiple clinical doses. *European Journal of Clinical Pharmacology*, 1980: 17: 135-143.
14. Shanks CA: Pharmacokinetics of non-depolarizing neuromuscular relaxants applied to calculation of bolus and infusion dosage regimes. *Anesthesiology*, 1986: 64: 72-86.
15. Stanski DR, et al: Pharmacokinetics and pharmacodynamics of d-tubocurarine during nitrous oxide-narcotic and halothane anesthesia in man. *Anesthesiology*, 1979: 51: 235-241.
16. Walker J, et al: Clinical pharmacokinetics of alcuronium in man. *European Journal of Clinical Pharmacology*, 1908: 17: 449-457.
17. Duvaldestein P, et al: Pancuronium pharmacokinetics in patients with liver cirrhosis. *British Journal of Anaesthesia*, 1978: 50: 1131-1135.
18. Lynam DP, et al: The pharmacodynamics and pharmacokinetics of vecuronium in patients anesthetized with isoflurane with normal renal function or with renal failure. *Anesthesiology*, 1988: 69: 227-231.
19. Ward S, Neill EAM: Pharmacokinetics of atracurium in acute hepatic failure (with acute renal failure). *British Journal of Anaesthesia*, 1983: 55: 1169-1172.
20. Mazoit J-X, et al: Pharmacokionetics of unchanged morphine in normal and cirrhotic subjects. *Anesthesiology*, 1987: 66: 293-298.
21. Gourlay GK, et al: A double-blind comparison of the efficacy of methadone and morphine in postoperative pain control. *Anesthesiology*, 1986: 64: 322-327.

22. Gourlay GK, et al: Pharmacokinetics and pharmacodynamics methadone during the perioperative period. *Anesthesiology*, 1982: 57: 458-467.

23. Mather LE, et al: Meperidine kinetics in man. Intravenous injection in surgical patients and volunteers. *Clinical Pharmacology & Therapeutics*, 1974: 17: 21-30.

24. Austin KL, et al: Relationship between blood meperidine concentrations and analgesic response. *Anesthesiology*, 1980: 53: 460-466.

25. Ehrnebo M, et al: Bioavailability and first-pass metabolism of pentazocine in man. *Clinical Pharmacology & Therapeutics*, 1977: 22: 888-892.

26. Berkowitz BA, et al: Relationship of pentazocine plasma levels to pharmacological activity in man. *Clinical Pharmacology & Therapeutics*, 1969: 10: 320-328.

27. Fischler M, et al: Pharmacokinetics of phenoperidine in anaesthetized patients undergoing general surgery. *British Journal of Anaesthesia*, 1985: 57: 872-876.

28. Milne L, et al: Plasma concentration and metabolism of phenoperidine in man. *British Journal of Anaesthesia*, 1980: 52: 537-539.

29. Haberer JP, et al: Fentanyl pharmacokinetics in anaesthetized patients with cirrhosis. *British Journal of Anaesthesia*, 1982: 54: 1267-1269.

30. Gourlay GK, et al: Fentanyl blood concentration-analgesc response relationship in the treatment of postoperative pain. *Anesthesia and Analgesia*, 1988: 67: 329-337.

31. Schüttler J, Stoekel H: Alfentanil (R39209) ein neues kurzwerkendes Opioid. Pharmakokinetik und erste klinische Erfahrungen. *Der Anaesthesist*, 1982: 31: 10-14.

32. O'Connor M, et al: Ventilatory depression during and after infusion of alfentanil in man. *British Journal of Anaesthesia*, 1983: 55: 217S-222S.

33. Hug CC, et al: Alfentanil plasma concentration versus effect relationships in cardiac surgical patients. *British Journal of Anaesthesia*, 1988: 61: 435-440.

34. Bovill JG, et al: The pharmacokinetics of sufentanil in surgical patients. *Anesthesiology*, 1984: 61: 502-506.

35. Goldfrank L, et al: A dosing nomogram for continuous infusion of intravenous naloxone. *Annals of Emergency Medicine*, 1986: 15: 566-570.

36. Clements JA, et al: The disposition of intravenous doxapram in man. *European Journal of Clinical Pharmacology*, 1979: 16: 411-416.

37. Robson RH, Prescott LF: A pharmacokinetic study of doxapram in patients and volunteers. *European Journal of Clinical Pharmacology*, 1978: 7: 81-87.

38. Hartvig P, et al: Pharmacokinetics of physostigmine after intravenous, intramuscular and subcutaneous administration in surgical patients. *Acta Anaesthesiologica Scandinavica*, 1986: 30: 177-182.

39. Klotz U, et al: Pharmacokinetics of the selective benzodiazepine antagonist Ro 15-1788 in man. *European Journal of Clinical Pharmacology*, 1984: 27: 115-117.

40. Klotz U: Drug interactions and clinical pharmacokinetics of flumazenil. *European Journal of Anaesthesiology*, 1988: supplement 2: 103-108.

41. Kanto J, Klotz U: ,(1988), Pharmacokinetic implications for the clinical use of atropine, scopolamine and glycopyrrolate. *Acta Anaesthesiologica Scandinavica*, 1988: 32: 69-78.

42. Calculated on the basis of the kinetic data and the dose-effect relationship in the article: Gravenstein JS, et al: Effects of atropine and scopolamine on the cardiovascular system in man. *Anesthesiology*, 1964: 25: 123-130.

43. Morris RB, et al: Pharmacokinetics of edrophonium and neostigmine when antagonizing d-tubocurarine neuromuscular blockade in man. *Anesthesiology*, 1981: 54: 399-402.

44. Cronnelly R, et al: Pyridostigmine kinetics with and without renal function. *Clinical Pharmacology & Therapeutics*, 1980: 28: 78-81.

45. Katz RL: Clinical neuromuscular pharmacology of pancuronium. *Anesthesiology*, 1971: 34: 550-556.

46. Rupp SM, et al: Neostigmine and edrophonium antagonism varying intensity neuromuscular blockade induced by atracurium, pancuronium, or vecuronium. *Anesthesiology*, 1986: 64: 711-717.
47. Hassan HA, Savarese JJ: Monitoring of neuromuscular function. *Anesthesiology*, 1976: 45: 216-249.
48. Viby-Mogensen J: Clinical assessment of neuromuscular transmission. *British Journal of Anaesthesia*, 1982: 54: 209-223.
49. O'Connor M, et al: Alfentanil infusions: Relationship between pharmacokinetics and pharmacodynamics in man. *European Journal of Anaesthesiology*, 1987: 4: 187-196.
50. Stanski DR, et al: Pharmacometrics: Pharmacodynamic modelling of thiopental anesthesia. *Journal of Pharmacokinetics and Biopharmaceutics*, 1984: 12: 223-240.
51. Arden JR, et al: Increased sensitivity to etomidate in the elderly: Initial distribution versus altered brain response. *Anesthesiology*, 1986: 65: 19-27.
52. Schüttler J, et al: Pharmacokinetic-dynamic modelling of diprivan. *Anesthesiology*, 1986: 65: A549.
53. Bührer M, et al: Comparative pharmacodynamics of midazolam and diazepam. *Anesthesiology*, 1988: 69: A642.
54. Scott JC, et al: EEG quantitfication of narcotic effect: The comparative pharmacodynamics of fentanyl and alfentanil. *Anesthesiology*, 1985: 62: 234-241.
55. Duvaldestin CJ, et al: Fazadinium and pancuronium: A pharmacodynamic study. *British Journal of Anaesthesia*, 1980: 52: 1209-1221.
56. Fisher DM, et al: Vecuronium kinetics and dynamics in anesthetized infants and children. *Clinical Pharmacology & Therapeutics*, 1985: 37: 402-406.
57. Cooke JE, Scott JC: Do fentanyl and sufentanil have the same pharmacodynamics? *Anesthesiology*, 1986: 65: A552.
58. Ghoneim MM, et al: Diazepam effects and kinetics in caucasians and orientals. *Clinical Pharmacology & Therapeutics*, 1981: 29: 749-756.
59. Reidenberg MM, et al: Relationships between diazepam dose, plasma level, age, and central nervous system depression. *Clinical Pharmacology & Therapeutics*, 1978: 23: 371-374.
60. Christensen JH, et al: Pharmacokinetics and pharmacodynamics of thiopentone. A comparison between young and elderly patients. *Anaesthesia*, 1982: 37: 399-404.
61. Bullingham RES, et al: Buprenorphine kinetics. *Clinical Pharmacology & Therapeutics*, 1980: 28: 667-672.
62. Parker CJR, Hunter JM: Plasma atracurium concentration-response relationship in patients anaesthetized with isoflurane. *British Journal of Anaesthesia*, 1988: 61: 105P-106P.

Appendix - B

Physical & Pharmacological Properties

This appendix is intended as a supplement to appendix-A. It provides physico-chemical and pharmacological data about the intravenous anesthetic drugs.

MW is the molecular weight expressed as grams/mole substance.

pKa is the pH at which the molecule is 50% ionized. The suffix "a" next to the pKa value in the table means that the molecule is an acid, and the suffix "b" next to the pKa value in the table means that the molecule is a base.

Protein binding is the percentage of the drug present in plasma which is bound to plasma proteins.

eryth/plasma is the erythrocyte/plasma concentration ratio or partition coefficient.

brain/plasma is the brain/plasma concentration ratio or partition coefficient.

fat/plasma is the fat or adipose tissue/plasma concentration ratio or partition coefficient.

muscle/plasma is the muscle/plasma concentration ratio or partition coefficient.

DRUG	MW (g/mole)	pKa	Protein binding (%)	eryth/ plasma	brain/ plasma	fat/ plasma	muscle/ plasma
INDUCTION AGENTS							
Thiopental	264.33	7.6a	80-84[21]	1[20]	1.4[1]	11[1]	1.5[1]
Methohexital	284.30	7.9a	73[21]			1-6[4]	
Hexobarbital	236.26						
Etomidate	244.28	4.24b	71-75[21]	1.0[18]			
Ketamine	237.74	7.5b	26[21]		6.5[6]		
Propofol	178.3	11.1b	98				
OPIATES							
Morphine	285.33	7.93b	35[21]		10[3]	0.8[8]	
Meperidine	247.34	8.5b	42-60[21]				
Methadone	345.9	9.26b	80[22]		0.7[13]		
Pentazocine	285.44	9.16b	65[22]				
Buprenorphine		8.51b	96[23]				
Phenoperidine	367.47						
Fentanyl	336.46	8.4b	84[21]	1.0[19]	7[2]	35[7]	3[7]
Alfentanil	471	6.5b	92[21]	0.14[19]	0.2[5]	0.2[5]	0.11[5]
Sufentanil	578.68	8.01b	92[21]				
ANALEPTICS & ANTAGONISTS							
Naloxone	327.37	7.82b			3.5[9]		
Doxapram	378.50						
Physostigmine	275.34						
Flumazenil	303.3	1.7b	50		3[12]		
MUSCLE RELAXANTS							
Succinylcholine	478.28						
Gallamine	891.56	>13b	0-70[21,24]	0.74[15]			
d-Tubocurarine	681.66	8.6b	43-51[21]			0[14]	0.16[14]
Alcuronium	737.80		40[21]				
Pancuronium	732.70	>13b	11-29[21]				
Vecuronium			30[21]				
Atracurium							
ANTICHOLINERGICS & ANTICHOLINESTERASES							
Atropine	289.38	9.8b			0.87[10,11]		
Neostigmine	334.39						
Pyridostigmine	261.14						
Edrophonium	246.15						
BENZODIAZEPINES							
Diazepam	284.76	3.3b	98-99[25]		2[16]	1[17]	
Lorazepam	321.16	1.3b	93				
Midazolam	325.80	6.2b	94[21]				

REFERENCES

1.   Price HL, et al: The uptake of thiopental by body tissues and its relation to the duration of narcosis. *Clinical Pharmacology & Therapeutics*, 1960: 1: 16-22.
2.   Ainslie SG, et al: Fentanyl concentrations in brain and serum during respiratory acid-base changes in the dog. *Anesthesiology*, 1979: 51: 293-297.
3.   Schulman DS, et al: Blood pH and brain uptake of ^{14}C-morphine. *Anesthesiology*, 1984: 61: 540-543.
4.   Brand L, et al: Physiologic disposition of methohexital man. *Anesthesiology*, 1963: 24: 331-335.
5.   Michiels M, et al,(1981), Plasma levels and tissue distribution of alfentanil (R39209) in the male Wistar rat after a ,single intravenous dose of 0.16 mg/kg. Janssen Research Products Information Report No. R39209/13.
6.   Cohen ML, et al: Distribution in the brain and metabolism of ketamine in the rat after intravenous administration. *Anesthesiology*, 1973: 39: 370-376.
7.   Hug CC, Murphy MR: Tissue redistribution of fentanyl and termination of its effects in rats. *Anesthesiology*, 1981: 55: 369-375.
8.   Hug CC, Murphy MR: Tissue distribution of morphine in rats. ?, 1984.
9.   Ngai SH, et al: Pharmacokinetics of naloxone in rats and in man: Basis for its potency and short duration of action. *Anesthesiology*, 1976: 44: 398-401.
10.   Proakis AG, Harris GB: Comparative penetration of glycopyrrolate and atropine across the blood-brain and placental barriers in anesthetized dogs. *Anesthesiology*, 1978: 48: 339 344.
11.   Kanto J, Klotz U: Pharmacokinetic implications for the clinical use of atropine, scopolamine and glycopyrrolate. *Acta Anaesthesiologica Scandinavica*, 1988: 32: 69-78.
12.   Klotz U: Drug interactions and clinical pharmcokinetics of flumazenil. *European Journal of Anaesthesiology*, 1988: supplement 2: 103-108.
13.   Robinson AE, Williams FM: The distribution of methadone in man. *Journal of Pharmacy and Pharmacology*, 1971: 23: 353-358.
14.   Cohen EN, et al: The distribution and fate of d-tubocurarine. *Journal of Pharmacology and Experimental Therapeutics*, 1965: 147: 120-129.
15.   Feldman SA, et al: The excretion of gallamine in the dog. *Anesthesiology*, 1969: 30: 593-598.
16.   Marcucci F, et al: Species difference in diazepam metabolism and anticonvulsant effect. *European Journal of Pharmacology*, 1968: 4: 467-470.
17.   Marcucci F, et al: Levels of diazepam in adipose tissue of rats, mice and man. *European Journal of Pharmacology*, 1968: 4: 464-466.
18.   Meuldermans WEG, Heykants JJP: The plasma protein binding and distribution of etomidate in dog, rat and human blood. *Arch. Int. Pharmacodyn.*, 1976: 221: 150-162.
19.   Bower S, Hull CJ: Comparative pharmacokinetics of fentanyl and alfentanil. *British Journal of Anaesthesia*, 1982: 54: 871-877.
20.   Morgan DJ, et al: Pharmacokinetics and plasma binding of thiopental. I. Studies in surgical patients. *Anesthesiology*, 1981: 54: 467-473.
21.   Wood M: Plasma drug binding: Implications for anesthesiologists. *Anesthesiology*, 1986: 65: 786-804.
22.   Vozeh S, et al: Pharmacokinetic drug data. *Clinical Pharmacokinetics*, 1988: 254-282.
23.   Heel RC, et al: Buprenorphine: A review of its pharmacological properties and therapeutic efficiency. *Drugs*, 1979: 17: 81-110.
24.   Ramzan MJ, et al: Clinical pharmacokinetics of the non-depolarizing muscle relaxants. *Clinical Pharmacokinetics*, 1981: 6: 25-60.

25. Kanto J, Klotz U: Intravenous benzodiazepines as anaesthetic agents: Pharmacokinetics and clinical consequences. *Acta Anaesthesiologica Scandinavica*, 1982: 26: 554-569.

Index
of Subjects

DEVELOPMENTS IN
CRITICAL CARE MEDICINE AND ANESTHESIOLOGY

1. O. Prakash (ed.): *Applied Physiology in Clinical Respiratory Care.* 1982
   ISBN 90-247-2662-X

2. M. G. McGeown: *Clinical Management of Electrolyte Disorders.* 1983
   ISBN 0-89838-559-8

3. T. H. Stanley and W. C. Petty (eds.): *New Anesthetic Agents, Devices and Monitoring Techniques.* Annual Utah Postgraduate Course in Anesthesiology. 1983
   ISBN 0-89838-566-0

4. P. A. Scheck, U. H. Sjöstrand and R. B. Smith (eds.): *Perspectives in High Frequency Ventilation.* 1983
   ISBN 0-89838-571-7

5. O. Prakash (ed.): *Computing in Anesthesia and Intensive Care.* 1983
   ISBN 0-89838-602-0

6. T. H. Stanley and W. C. Petty (eds.): *Anesthesia and the Cardiovascular System.* Annual Utah Postgraduate Course in Anesthesilogy. 1984
   ISBN 0-89838-626-8

7. J. W. van Kleef, A. G. L. Burm and J. Spierdijk (eds.): *Current Concepts in Regional Anaesthesia.* 1984
   ISBN 0-89838-644-6

8. O. Prakash (ed.): *Critical Care of the Child.* 1984
   ISBN 0-89838-661-6

9. T. H. Stanley and W. C. Petty (eds.): *Anesthesiology: Today and Tomorrow.* Annual Utah Postgraduate Course in Anesthesiology. 1985
   ISBN 0-89838-705-1

10. H. Rahn and O. Prakash (eds.): *Acid-base Regulation and Body Temperature.* 1985
    ISBN 0-89838-708-6

11. T. H. Stanley and W. C. Petty (eds.): *Anesthesiology 1986.* Annual Utah Postgraduate Course in Anesthesiology. 1986
    ISBN 0-89838-779-5

12. S. de Lange, P. J. Hennis and D. Kettler (eds.): *Cardiac Anaesthesia.* Problems and Innovations. 1986
    ISBN 0-89838-794-9

13. N. P. de Bruijn and F. M. Clements: *Transesophageal Echocardiography.* With a contribution by R. Hill. 1987
    ISBN 0-89838-821-X

14. G. B. Graybar and L. L. Bready (eds.): *Anesthesia for Renal Transplantation.* 1987
    ISBN 0-89838-837-6

15. T. H. Stanley and W. C. Petty (eds.): *Anesthesia, the Heart and the Vascular System.* Annual Utah Postgraduate Course in Anesthesiology. 1987
    ISBN 0-89838-851-1

16. D. Reis Miranda, A. Williams and Ph. Loirat (eds.): *Management of Intensive Care.* Guidelines for Better Use of Resources. 1990
    ISBN 0-7923-0754-2

17. T. H. Stanley (ed.): *What's New in Anesthesiology.* Annual Utah Postgraduate Course in Anesthesiology. 1988
    ISBN 0-89838-367-6

18. G. M. Woerlee: *Common Perioperative Problems and the Anaesthetist.* 1988
    ISBN 0-89838-402-8

19. T. H. Stanley and R. J. Sperry (eds.): *Anesthesia and the Lung.* Annual Utah Postgraduate Course in Anesthesiology. 1989
    ISBN 0-7923-0075-0

20. J. De Castro, J. Meynadier and M. Zenz: *Regional Opioid Analgesia.* Physiopharmacological Basis, Drugs, Equipment and Clinical Application. 1990
    ISBN 0-7923-0162-5

21. J. F. Crul (ed.): *Legal Aspects of Anaesthesia.* 1989
    ISBN 0-7923-0393-8

DEVELOPMENTS IN
CRITICAL CARE MEDICINE AND ANESTHESIOLOGY

KLUWER ACADEMIC PUBLISHERS – DORDRECHT / BOSTON / LONDON